THE WESTERN
BOOK OF DEATH

by Adriana Balthazar, MD; PhD

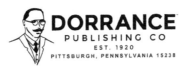

DORRANCE
PUBLISHING CO
EST. 1920
PITTSBURGH, PENNSYLVANIA 15238

Dorrance Publishing Co
585 Alpha Drive
Suite 103
Pittsburgh, PA 15238
Visit our website at *www.dorrancebookstore.com*

ISBN: 978-1-4809-2756-8
eISBN: 978-1-4809-2894-7

CONTENTS

INTRODUCTION

Of the various resource books about death and dying, produced by humanity during different historical periods, one of the most ancient is *The Egyptian Book of the Dead,* or *Pert em hru* ("The Coming Forth by Day" or "Manifestation in the light"). It is a compilation of texts from several different times in the history of Egypt, beginning in 3100 BC. This book contains hymns as well as magic words of power and procedures used mainly in the ceremonies performed at the time of death and as inscriptions in the tombs, it served the purpose of leading the soul toward a joyful union with God.

Another well known book about the process of death is *The Tibetan Book of the Dead,* or *Bardo Thodol,* ("Liberation Through Understanding in the Between"), produced by Padma Sambhava during the eighth century. *The Tibetan Book of the Dead* is used before, during, and after the moment of death, to help individuals die in the best possible manner, by reminding and guiding them to identify postmortem stages in order to attain liberation, or at least a good rebirth. Its teachings and instructions also provide the living with knowledge about the death process, preparing them for it and encouraging them not to hold onto departing individuals.

The former two books depict the soul's pilgrimage after physical death, through distinct stages, providing prayers and instructions to help guide the departed one, and discussing death, resurrection, and rebirth.

Within the Judeo/Christian tradition, although a book of the dead as such does not exists, the stories contained in the first six books of the Old Testament, can be considered a kind of Hebrew book of the dead, as they tell about the challenges of the human soul on its transit through different worlds and contain hidden messages that seem to reflect the progression of the soul through the cycles of birth, life in the material world, death, life in the inner world, and reincarnation. In addition, many Christian texts about death and dying, known as *"Ars Moriendi"*, were written in Europe, especially during the Middle Ages. In many of these literary works, the stance of facing and favorably receiving death is encouraged.

Further, there are also *The Mayan Book of the Dead,* or *Popol Vuh* ("The Ballgame in the Underworld") and *The Nahuatl Book of the Dead* (the story of Quetzalcoatl or the Plumed Serpent) that symbolically depict the journey, trials, and evolution of the human soul in the underworld, as well as they refer to resurrection, rebirth, and the eventual transformation of humans into celestial beings.

Today, although these books of the dead are still available to us, it is difficult for the majority of people in the occidental world to relate to them, understand them, and use them properly. Therefore, the purpose of *The Western Book of Death is* to provide accessible information about the process of death, the journey of the human soul, and the cycles of life, death, intermission, and reincarnation. Thus, individuals will have less fear of death, will make the subject no longer a taboo, and will be able to better prepare for the inevitable stages of their evolution.

CHAPTER I

The Process of Death: Overview

Death is the process by which an individual soul departs, leaving behind its outer garment of flesh (the physical body) and eventually, also the lower subtle bodies (emotional and lower mental bodies), and moves from one realm of existence to another. This may happen either unconsciously or consciously. Death implies nothing more than losing the three lower vehicles of consciousness which we carry only for a while, during each living experience on Earth, and which are not who we really are at a deeper level.

Dying is like crossing a threshold that leads to a new life, with new conditions and expanded consciousness in another plane of existence. In other words, we continue living in another wave length world, our focus of attention has veered in a different direction, and a shift in consciousness has taken place.

Death is brought about by the will of the soul/spirit, which controls matter. It offers the individual soul partial liberation and rest from the denser dimension of matter, accompanied by an increased vibratory speed of our being, and marks the end of the soul's opportunities to evolve within a particular body and during a specific life on Earth.

Death is an interlude that provides the possibilities for reflection, assessment, integration, and renovation, prior to the undertaking of a new life period on the outer world, or reincarnation.

Mastery of the art of dying is accomplished when the individual is capable of consciously and wisely returning the lower bodies and the soul to their respective sources on due time.

The science that studies the phenomena of death and the psychological mechanisms for coping with them is called *Thanatology.*

DEATH AS AN ILLUSION

What we call death is only part of a continuum of life. Our life is an ever flowing, unbroken stream of conscious existence, whether we are on a planet or not. Thus, if we acquire knowledge about that which we call death, we are really learning more about life. Both, birth and death are intertwined and parts of a process of spiritual evolution. Both signify passing through a door toward a new beginning. Therefore, death as we generally understand it, can be considered one of the biggest illusions of the material plane.

Nothing really dies. There is but changes in form and activity, rather than dying. For instance, the human physical body never truly dies, for its atoms, after physical death and the withdrawal of the spirit aspect (soul) that kept them together, disperse and return to their source, in order to form something else later.

When we are born on our planet, we lose the memory of our previous lives, in order to adjust to the dense, illusory physical world of duality. In this world, then, our consciousness is veiled, and we perceive things through the lens of our physical senses, which are bombarded by interminable stimuli, and that, in a way, mask our connection to the unseen worlds. However, this impermanent part of our journey is necessary for further evolution and growth.

What happens is that usually we erroneously identify ourselves as being only a physical body, believing exclusively in the experience of and information from the physical sense organs. From this perspective, yes, we disappear; we end our existence at the time of the so called death. But, we are not the appearance of the physical body. Our true identity lies beyond the material form. We are pure spirit and consciousness, that which animates our body, that which is the master of the body, that which is eternal.

Death as we generally understand it, is a concept, an idea which is rooted in ignorance and illusion. We may say then, that we misunderstand death. Since the human mind in general believe that death is something terminal and final, the human mind pronounces itself against death and does not want to deal with it, often acting as if death were a taboo subject. This means that we are avoiding a very important part of life and we are separating that which is inseparable and intimately connected: life and death.

Once we come to live here on Earth we learn that amidst all the uncertainties and impermanent conditions of this life there is just one thing that is certain, and that is the moment of the so called death. From a deeper perspective, death is considered as a change of state, as the termination of a particular form of something. Then, what else is life but a series of such changes and transformation, a sequence of infinitesimal small deaths? In reality, we are "dying" to something every single second of our lives. Thus, in a particular way, we are quite familiar with death. Cells in our physical body are constantly being renewed, so that the body is not the same from minute to minute, it is transformed (dies) millions of times. And so it happens with the emotional and mental bodies.

From the same perspective, each time we exhale, we die; each time we inhale, we live. Each time we let go of the past, we die. Each time we go to sleep, we die to the physical plane and function in some other realm or dream landscape. In addition, with regard to the larger cycles of life, we must realize that we have died many times, each life period on a planet, and will continue to do so until we complete our planetary evolution.

Death is a <u>process</u> which is one with that of life. Death is the joyous activity of <u>Spirit ever and ever entering into life.</u> There is only <u>continuity.</u> There is <u>no death.</u>

THE FEAR OF DEATH

In western cultures, people generally have such a fear of death that the subject is regarded almost as a taboo.

We fear death for a variety of reasons. First, perhaps the most important reason is our ignorance. We do not know life in depth and consequently don't understand death. We are not afraid of death because of the fact itself but because death is unknown to us. We do not know what will happen or not happen at the moment of death and thereafter. Unless we learn to live in the present without fears and acknowledge that life is eternal, we will continue fearing death.

In addition, our insistence on viewing things as compartmentalized, or in terms of dualities, and thus seeing life and death as two different things provokes anxiety and fear of death. In other words, our tendency not to view life and death as a continuum results in this fear.

Another reason for our fear of death is rooted in our identification with the physical body and the excessive importance we give it. When we see this material form decaying and know it will eventually disappear after death, we certainly experience apprehension and have difficulty facing it. We fear the termination of the self. But our life does not depend on the functioning of a physical body, which is only a transitory vehicle in this material realm. Thus we must learn to live in complete consciousness as souls while here on Earth. From this perspective, there is no death, and we are part of the force we call God. Instead, there is eternal life and a ceaseless evolution of consciousness.

Our dread of death may also originate with our fear of being alone as at birth and separated from all that which is familiar to us, including leaving loved ones behind. However, any comparison of the circumstances of birth and death is unjustified. At birth the individual soul is confined to a restrictive body, incapable of taking care of itself, and surrounded by a totally foreign environment inhabited by strangers, since there is no recollection of past links. However, during and after the transition of death, we are not alone. We may be surrounded by those we have known on Earth, as well as by guides, angels, and teachers from other realms. In addition, we are clearly aware of loved ones left behind still on the physical plane and can tune in to their emotions and thoughts since they are always present within our hearts, regardless of whether both of us are on Earth or in another world. The feeling of losing someone by either our death or theirs is merely based on an idea, and the suffering caused by it originates only in the attachment to the physical form of manifestation.

One more reason for our fear of death is due to emotions instilled in us by some religious teachings that emphasize such concepts as "the day of judgment", "the punishment of God", and "hell". But there is no punishment as we understand it. The whole of Creation is animated and kept together in cohesion by a great Law of Love.

Finally, our fear of death can be fueled by unconscious reactions to a past life experience of violent death.

In summary, we may say that the fear of death is mostly based on:

- Ignorance.
- Separating death from life.
- Identifying with and clinging to the physical body.
- Assuming that we are going to be alone in the midst of strangers and unfamiliar environments.
- The thought of leaving loved ones behind or of being left behind.

- Doubts about our immortality.
- Accepting erroneous beliefs about "judgment", "punishment" and "hell".
- Strong impressions on the subconscious mind of a violent death in a past life.

The tremendous fear induced by old concepts about death can be transcended by deeply understanding the following:

- <u>Death is a significant part of life</u> within a ceaseless and continuous process of spiritual evolution.
- <u>There is no separation</u> from anything.
- <u>There is only life.</u>
- <u>Birth and death are sacred portals</u> through which we must pass during our journey. We must learn to move beyond the common concepts that we now hold about birth and death.
- <u>Death is a transition.</u> Going from life to death is like moving from one room to another, from one city to another.
- <u>Nothing ever dies.</u> There is but continuity of manifestation in different forms.
- <u>We are Soul/Spirit</u> and as such, we can never be destroyed.
- <u>We are multidimensional beings,</u> capable of focusing our consciousness on any plane of existence at will so that while living on Earth we can be in touch with other dimensions provided we can master the abilities to do this.
- <u>We are not only a physical body</u>.
- <u>We are never alone.</u>
- <u>There is neither punishment nor condemnation.</u>

Also, for us to lose the fear of death it would be a great help if:

- <u>We acquire information</u> about the process of dying, the near-death experience phenomenon, and encounters with deceased people.
- <u>We learn to live entirely in the present moment</u>. This places our consciousness within the eternal flow of Spirit and helps keep us from separating that which is inseparable; making us more aware of life as a continuum.

- <u>We become ready for change and transformation,</u> not being attached to physical forms.
- <u>We work with our dreams consistently</u> and become familiar with dream landscapes, thus we can gain awareness of other realms that will be transited after death.
- <u>We practice daily meditation.</u> In such state we open doors to higher consciousness, discover that we are limitless and not confined to a dense physical body, and perceive the unbroken continuity of life.

Fears, doubts, and anxiety prevent us from really living. When we eliminate our fear of death, we truly experience freedom and well-being. As we clear our minds from past conditioning and begin to better understand the process of dying and the concept of other dimensions, we gain a new attitude toward the great transition we call death that incorporates acceptance, peace, and joy.

THE TRANSITION OF DEATH

The right time for death is basically decided by the soul, whether the individual is conscious or unconscious of it. After physical death happens, a dissociation of the lower bodies follows (physical, etheric, emotional, lower mental).The energy thread connecting the soul to the lower bodies separates from them and is absorbed by the soul carrying within itself the imprints of the most elevated aspirations of the individual while the imprints of inferior deeds remain dispersed in space until the time comes when they are magnetically attracted to the new personality of the individual as part of karmic debts and prior to reincarnation. The lower bodies then dissolve, returning their component elements to their source and to the conditions and settings that psycho-magnetically attract them, and become part of something else.

During the intervening period between two Earth lives, the physical life-atoms that constitute a physical body may transmigrate through the other kingdoms of nature (mineral, vegetal, animal) and also through the human kingdom, always following the Law of Attraction/Repulsion, that is, attracted by entities with similar vibratory rate, and repulsed by unlike vibrations.

The Etheric body is the vehicle for *prana* which is the life energy used and directed by the soul in order to enliven the lower bodies that make possible its manifestation on Earth. When the soul departs from the physical body and this begins to disintegrate, each physical atom leaves with its individual charge of *prana* to form new associations. Another part of the vital energy contained within

6

the etheric body leaves with the soul and the residual portion returns to the universal pool of energy.

After the soul departs the physical body and is temporarily free from its dense vesture it carries three permanent atoms (physical, emotional, mental). The permanent atoms consist of the coded information reflecting the total learning and evolution undergone by the individual at the physical, emotional, and mental levels and during all previous lives.

The soul is then in the astral realm corresponding to the experiences of the individual in the recent life on Earth and will remain for some time enshrouded with the emotional body depending upon the character and magnitude of the yearnings and desires of the individual. Afterward, the emotional body is abandoned as well, and the astral shell eventually dissipates into astral substance; then, in due time the soul also leaves behind the lower mental body to dissolve onto mental substance. Thus after the transition of death, the soul goes through a period of releasing all attachments related to matter, desires, and habits, while learning and education continue beyond the realms of the world of physical matter.

Ultimately, the soul endures clothed in the causal body, an envelope of high mental energy, until the time for its next reincarnation is due. The period between two incarnations is called "Devachan" in Buddhist tradition. We may say that each time we die we discard layers, like taking off old clothes, while our immortal Self passes into more elevated states of consciousness.

This release from the physical body happens unconsciously while we are alive each time we go to sleep. However, it can also be accomplished consciously and at will, a practice known as astral travel, or astral projection. In such a state we function through the subtler astral and mental bodies in a foreign dimension and we are completely aware of it.

When the soul is in the lighter, freer state of the disembodied condition, the restrictions that characterize physical existence are gone, and with no physical brain the mind is liberated from the concept of linear time (past, present, future). In this new condition time as we understand it does not exists. However, after death we find that our individual essence and our free will remain and the veil of illusions still exists, although it is thinner than when we donned garments of flesh.

The condition we find ourselves in after death depends on what we have done during our lives on Earth, regarding desires, thoughts, aspirations, choices, and deeds. Each of us is the only responsible one for our own state posterior to death, as we are during life on the material plane. The most important factor that determines our condition after death is our capacity to love.

Once in the afterlife, our souls *are* the only judges of our past deeds and use of the previous life opportunities. On the other side, there are no masks concealing our real selves. There we are openly seen for what we really are and we are grouped together with like- minded souls.

During the transition of death we are not alone. Helper spirits are present whether they are guides, teachers, friends, or loved ones. Thus, when facing the changes of death, we may ask for assistance from spiritual guides and teachers, as well as from individuals left behind in the physical world. In fact, the individuals who undergo the transformation of death are at first very aware of the persons left behind on Earth, although they do not experience missing them in the true sense of the word. Being in a new world of existence and higher learning, they become primarily preoccupied with participating in new activities, especially during the stages immediately following death. According to Buddhist tradition the places where we find ourselves after death are known as "Bardos", which are not physical locations but states of consciousness.

The more we develop spiritually we identify ourselves mainly with the soul and the more we are able to open ourselves to love, compassion, and transformation in all conditions, the easier our transition onto death will be and the higher the consciousness we will experience afterwards. By contrast, the more we are self centered; attached to material things and pleasures brought about by the physical senses, or the presence of other human beings, or the more barbarous deeds we commit, more earthbound we will be after death, as the soul remains so engrossed with its previous life activities that cannot let go of them and instead stay close to the physical places and persons of the former life, insisting in getting involved with chores of terrestrial living.

Commonly children experience the easiest transition at death, since they are still more in tune with the spiritual realms they just left and have not been immersed in the material existence long enough to develop the kind of attachments, misconceptions, and fears adults do.

Generally, those individuals who are yet undeveloped as human beings experience the process of death as a kind of unconscious sleeping or forgetting, because their minds are not awakened enough to allow them much awareness.

After death, moderately developed individuals continue existing in the same state of consciousness, with the same inclinations and interests, and their new circumstances are an extension of their former physical lives.

Individuals who are highly evolved spiritually are totally lucid and in a realm of high learning, communication, and service.

The period that souls require to become accustomed to their new environments after death varies according to the abilities of individuals, the circumstances of death and the degree of attachment to memories from the recent life on Earth. The process of adaptation is easier for people who are open minded, ready to accept changes, and more difficult for those who cling to rigid and narrow belief systems or do not believe in an afterlife, who may endure disoriented and confused as earth bound entities.

When the time is right, the soul prepares itself for a new terrestrial journey or reincarnation, carrying the three permanent atoms which shall serve as seeds for the formation of brand new lower bodies (mental, emotional, physical) which will constitute the new personality in the coming life on Earth. One life time on Earth is only a transient experience which is part of the continuum of eternal Life.

The fact that the soul, while incarnated, is enveloped with the lower bodies contributes significantly to the illusion we experience. During life on Earth we forget past lives and thus lose awareness of the continuity of life unless we consciously develop sufficiently spiritually and become totally awakened.

In conclusion, the soul periodically leaves its natural condition and dives into physical life with the purpose of gaining experiences through the physical senses and then returns progressively enriched by those experiences. Thus, our planet Earth serves as a needed school, where learning to remember who we are and spiritual growth take place.

Each reincarnation represents the continuation of certain inclinations, qualities, and connections pertaining to the individual who is going through a long trajectory of evolution, except that each life period occurs in the context of different arrangements and thus is perceived by us as a totally new and dissociated life.

The uncountable short cycles of planetary material life in linear time/space ,with the illusion of separation, followed by death and return to the unseen spiritual worlds, are only to qualify the soul for ever higher levels of awareness and existence. The process of death is then a limited portion of a ceaseless current of eternal life.

THE IMPORTANCE OF HOW WE ENCOUNTER DEATH

The transition of death takes a different form for various individuals, depending on their degree of awareness and realization during their lifetime on Earth. However, generally we may experience the passage of death in one of two ways, either consciously or unconsciously, both of which have profound effects upon us and the immediate circumstances in which we find ourselves.

The most usual kind of experience is dying unconsciously, whether death was anticipated or not. In these circumstances individuals are ignorant of the process of death and die not prepared for it at all. For them death is experienced almost like a forced expulsion of the soul from a deteriorating physical body. This results in instinctive, mechanical reactions, such as shock, confusion, and fear, especially if dying individuals are alone at the moment of death. This manner of dying leads the soul to retract away from Light encounters and to a narrow state of consciousness with surroundings that reflect it. The soul does not merge with Light due to inability to let go of concepts of limitation, negative patterns, and fear.

Individuals who are cognizant of the process of death and prepared, die consciously. They are able to make the transition from the material plane to the various inner planes totally aware, in a fearless, relaxed, and joyous manner. Such a way of dying allows for further consciousness expansion, a fuller encounter with the Light and possibly a total merging with it that could result in enlightenment, or liberation. Consequently, dying consciously has potent, positive effects not only for individuals but also for humanity and life in general.

Another very important factor that determines conditions at death is the nature of the thoughts we entertain at that very moment. These are decisive due to the fact that a little further into the death process our individuality shall be drawn toward the conditions reflecting the qualities of those thoughts which are projected and eventually create our inner reality in the afterlife and go as far as influencing the process of reincarnation and conditions in the next lifetime on Earth.

Consequently, if last thoughts of individuals are positive, of the Light or Spirit, their consciousness expands to corresponding states and circumstances in the afterlife period and also later results in positive conditions for the next rebirth on the planet. Sustaining elevated thoughts at the moment of death may open the possibility of even achieving enlightenment. Conversely, if the last thoughts of dying persons are negative — due to ignorance, shock, or fear — these will cause corresponding conditions in the afterlife period and also later at rebirth.

From the former paragraphs we can see clearly that the situations and the character of the afterlife conditions and even of the next terrestrial life are strongly linked to the very moment of death in the previous life. Thus the quality of the moment of death has tremendous importance due to the fact that it brings the possibility for growth in consciousness toward awareness of our unity with God and even for enlightenment, which occurs when the substance of our consciousness, like a mirror, perfectly reflects the Pure Reality of Light. This is possible only when the mirror is crystal clear, free from the turmoil of thoughts, emotions, and afflictions of the physical body, enabling us to recognize the Light as the Reality of ourselves — what it is referred to as Self-realization.

OUR ATTITUDE TOWARD DEATH

Currently our attitude toward death is often one of fear and avoidance due to our ignorance, doubts, emphasis on the material part of life, and attachments to physical forms.

We frequently try to interfere with the natural process of death by clinging desperately to our physical body, even when it is no longer able to serve its purpose and thus keeps the soul imprisoned when, in reality the soul is trying to be free because it certainly knows the time has come for relinquishing the physical body and entering into a period of integrating experiences and information gathered during the recent lifetime.

Fortunately, the evolutionary course of humanity will lead to a future time when individuals shall be living as spiritual beings, with perfect knowledge of the death process and prescribed term of an incarnation and will be ready to joyously withdraw from the physical vehicle when its service is no longer needed. At this time, individuals will know with certainty that the physical body is only an instrument through which the Divine Plan is temporarily served and even have the ability to lengthen or shorten the periods of planetary life at will, in accordance with their awareness of the purpose of a particular lifetime. Ultimately, there will be no death as we know it, just a voluntary departure from a physical body catalyzed by awareness of the stages of evolution.

HOW DO WE KNOW ABOUT DEATH?

We know about death through various sources, including:

- The teachings of Avatars and Prophets.
- The teachings of spiritual teachers, and philosophers such as Plato and Emanuel Swedenborg.

- Information from psychics and channels, who receive it from disincarnate teachers and ordinary beings.
- Having had out-of-body experiences (astral traveling) and remembering it.
- Working with our dreams and practicing lucid dreaming.
- Practicing deep meditation.
- Information obtained through the study of mythological stories.
- Information we have received ourselves through personal communication with deceased individuals.
- Information provided by the investigators in the field of near-death experiences, death, and reincarnation such as William Welch, Peter Fenwick, Dr Elizabeth Kubler-Ross, Dr Ian Stevenson, Dr Jim Tucker, Dr Pem Ven Lomo, Dr Jeffrey Long, Dr Bruce Greyson, and Dr Raymond Moody.
- Information provided in books such as The Tibetan Book of the Dead, The Egyptian Book of the Dead, The Hebrew Book of the Dead, The Popol Vuh, and others.
- Information available in the Scriptures — if we know how to discover it.

THE NEAR-DEATH EXPERIENCE

Under this name are described cases in which people undergo clinical death pronounced by professional staff and then, due to resuscitation procedures or not, reenter the body and come back to physical life.

The near-death experiences constitute one of the most unshakable proofs that we possess of the continuation of life following death. Many thousands of individuals of all ages, sexes, races, religions, and nationalities have had such experiences, well documented by numerous medical doctors, psychiatrists, psychologists, and investigators of the subject. This experience may be considered as a universal phenomenon that takes place in the astral plane of existence when the soul of the individual in question is out of the physical body.

According to research the following are the most commonly mentioned stages of this experience and the sequence in which they occur:

- Individuals hear the professional staff pronouncing their death.
- Thereafter, they hear a buzzing or ringing noise.

- They feel they are traveling along a dim tunnel at an extraordinary speed. The sensation is like been forcefully propelled.
- They realize then that they are in the vicinity of their own physical body but outside, observing it in a detached manner, usually, witnessing the resuscitation techniques being performed on their bodies.
- They find themselves in a state of emotional perplexity, although they do not feel the pain of the physical body.
- They become calmer and better adapted to their unfamiliar condition.
- They discover that they still possess a body, although one with different characteristics and abilities than the physical body they exited.
- They see, and some times, converse with others coming to receive and help them to become more alert and calm about the new circumstances surrounding them. The new comers could be already deceased friends or relatives, angels, religious figures, or spiritual guides.
- They are sometimes shown different locations and scenarios such as historical places, planets belonging to other solar systems, other dimensions of existence and also schools existing at those levels. Other times, they receive revelations, or are shown events of the future. From these descriptions it becomes evident that the experimenters of a near-death phenomenon may visit many different levels of the other world and some of these conditions are very similar to those on Earth, while others are very different. The majority of near-death experience subjects describe positive and very pleasant experiences, as "heavens", while a minority experience fearful and negative situations, as "hells".
- They encounter a powerful Being of Light who communicates with them mentally, transmitting intense warmth, love, understanding, healing, and protection. This Being may appear as an immense, resplendent, blinding, pulsating, colorless glowing sphere, one that has yellow, gold, and white colors, or a black depth shining with a shade of purple that radiates an indescribable sense of peace. Individuals feel embraced by this Being of Light, becoming one with its pulsations, and experience that all their doubts about the oneness of the entire Creation are dissipated. They lose their individuality and at the same time know who they are — an extension of the Primal Force. This sense of knowing and intense feeling causes them to experience a state of extreme joy and elation.

- The Light Being asks a question related to values and love in life, causing individuals to deeply assess their lives on Earth. Simultaneously, they undergo a life review, which may occur either in the form of a quick viewing of the main events in their lives — like glimpses of some parts of a film strip —, or as a complete, panoramic sequence of events from beginning to end, including sometimes the moment of their birth and even further back, the instant of their conception. This review consists not only of seeing images of events but also reliving these events feeling and understanding the consequences of behavior and deeds while alive, the reasons for certain circumstances, and the impact of actions, thoughts, and intentions on others.
- The individuals reviewing their lives are the sole judges of themselves and without the shadow of a doubt know what they did during life on Earth in terms of learning and loving. This life review functions as a potent catalyst for future transformation in the lives of those experiencing them when they return to physical existence.
- Everything around the individuals turns brilliant and vibrant, and they feel more alive than during their lives on Earth
- In most of the cases the individuals feel immersed in a sea of calmness, love, and felicity.
- The individuals eventually come to a boundary, which could appear in the shape of a barrier, a line, a river, a path, or simply as fog. At this point, they are telepathically told to return to earthly life, that this is not their moment of death.
- The individuals often oppose going back, due to the feelings of joy, peace, and love they have already experienced on the other side. Nevertheless, they reconnect with their physical bodies and reappear on the stage of terrestrial life.

After Effects of the Near-Death Experience

Everyone who has gone through a near-death experience testifies to consequences for their lives, especially its significant effects on their approach to life and death, and their relation with others. Such experiences always act as catalysts for individuals to make fundamental changes in their lives.

The physical and psychological effects of having a near-death experience can be summed up as follows:

Effects on the Physical Level
-   Feeling invigorated, as if having received a powerful energy current.
-   Experiencing an enhanced sensitivity to sounds and lights.
-   Development of extrasensory faculties.
-   Changes in the natural body cycles (reversal of the clock mechanism).
-   Having multiple perceptions with one sense, such as hearing a color, or seeing a sound.
-   Experiencing low blood pressure.
-   Changes in the digestive system and intolerance to certain foods.
-   Changes in the nervous system, body chemistry, and functioning of the brain.
-   Intolerance to regular medications.

Effects on the Psychological Level
-   Difficulty in describing the experience due to the limitations of our language.
-   Stimulation of intellectual faculties.
-   Augmentation of the intuitive faculty.
-   Arousal of creativity.
-   Diminished stress.
-   Sense of freedom from the restrictions of linear time.
-   Loss of the fear of death.
-   Decreased preoccupation with materialistic aims and increased spiritual orientation.
-   Feeling more loving and compassionate.
-   Becoming charismatic, with a glowing appearance.
-   Change of occupation to one more involved with service to healing others.
-   Increased and clear understanding of an unfinished mission on Earth.
-   Clearer comprehension of the Divine Plan.
-   Steadfast resolution to make changes that will lead to a positive social contribution to the well-being of humanity.

The Near-Death Experience in Cases of Attempted Suicide

According to research, individuals who have had a near-death experience as a result of attempted suicide later realize that their attempt was useless and did not help them to resolve the circumstances from which they wanted to escape. Such individuals recount finding themselves within the grips of exactly the same circumstances on the other side during the interlude spent outside their physical bodies.

The Empathic Near-Death Experience

An empathic near-death experience is one lived by individuals who are very close to dying loved ones, are present at the moment of their deaths and thus co-experience and share the transition of death with their beloved ones, even accompanying them momentarily to the other side. This is the result of pure empathy.

People who have experience such phenomena claim to have seen the tunnel, felt the presence of already deceased beings, and seen the Light, or even left their bodies and move together with the dying ones for some time before returning to their physical vehicles. The effects of this kind of experience on the current lives of the persons who went through them are the same as those for others experiencing the near-death phenomenon in different ways.

CHAPTER II

Stages fo the Process of Death:
Stage 1 - Preliminary Stage
Stage 2 - Restoration Stage

Death marks the end of a cycle — a period of life, as one kind of expression, is followed by a period of death, as another kind of expression — and follows the universal Law of Pendulum, also known as Law of Rhythm or Law of Cycles, under which equilibrium is attained, as well as the universal Law of Attraction, which represents the manifestation of the second Divine Aspect of Love/Wisdom.

Thus the soul, which has completed its purpose for a particular life period, shifts its focus away from the physical world toward the inner worlds, and consciously brings this incarnation to an end through its will and its increased receptivity to the power of Spirit, which at this point overrides the attraction of matter. At the same time another magnetic force, the elemental force of the Earth's spirit, acts on the physical body provoking the release and return of its substance to its source. It is the soul then that signals the personality of the individual and the mind receives the order of departure transmitting it to the brain, where the consciousness thread of energy is anchored, then to the heart, where the life thread of energy is held. The physical body acknowledges the signal and begins to dissolve, deferring to the power of the soul.

The process of death continues with the actual separation of the subtler bodies from the physical body and results in the following:

- The etheric body is dismembered and loses its magnetic attraction for the physical body, freeing the soul. A minimal amount of the etheric substance which constituted the etheric body remains within the physical body to provide prana, or vital force, to the physical atoms, which eventually pass to constitute new forms. Another, larger portion of the etheric substance, is discarded by the departing soul as the shell of the former etheric body. This shell slowly disintegrates, returning its atoms to the primordial ethers and its charge of prana to the universal reservoir of life force. A third portion of etheric substance, which contains all the karmic and evolutionary information about the individual, endures with the departing soul. Thus after the soul exits, the life force that formerly enlivened or animated the physical body ceases.
- The entities known as Divas and Builders, who contributed to the construction and maintenance of the physical body through the manipulation of pranic energy, withdraw, since the attraction of the will of the soul exists no longer.
- The entities whose purpose is the destruction of forms dissolve the physical body. The physical atoms are scattered, taking their portion of prana, and return to the atomic pool of matter to be used in new combinations. Thus, substance and energy remain, while forms do not last.

With the separation of the etheric body from the dense physical body, that part of the silver cord (magnetic energy thread) that links the physical body to the emotional, or astral body breaks, completely liberating from the physical body the etheric body with the soul, which remains enshrouded in the astral and lower mental vehicles and then discards the etheric body.

Stages of the Process of Death
In this chapter and the following (chapter III) a detailed discussion of the process of death is presented, which helps to clarify the preceding general overview of the process. The whole process of death comprises four different stages:

1) Preliminary stage, prior to the moment of death.
2) Restoration stage, the moment of death.
3) Shedding stage, immediately following the moment of death.

4) Assimilation stage, later on the journey through the inner worlds. The last two stages (three and four) take place during the intermission between two planetary life periods.

1) Preliminary Stage

All people know unconsciously when death is coming, simply because the soul knows and commands it, and some are consciously aware, in occasions verbally expressing it. In many cases, such people are warned of their impending death through dreams or signs during daily life. This knowledge of imminent death, conscious or unconscious may lead to changes in behavior or normal routine months prior to the occurrence of death. For example, they may immediately take care of unfinished personal matters; reevaluate activities and goals in their lives; feel the need to contact and see persons who are special to them or resolve conflicts with others; shift focus to spiritual concerns rather than material ones and exhibit certain wisdom and a resplendent appearance in anticipation of approaching the inner worlds. It appears that at this point the right brain hemisphere activity predominates.

During the days prior to death, individuals may exhibit modifications of needs and change in the gestures or the language they use to express themselves, including talking in a symbolic, or metaphoric manner. Other common experiences of individuals close to dying are visions of already dead relatives, loved ones, or celestial beings, or symbolic visions, such as fire in a mirror or dream like scenarios. There is also alteration in the colors of the individual's energy fields, or auras, which appear as if veiled by smoke, giving them a grayish tint, a change that can be perceived by those who have developed astral vision.

Several hours before death the individuals might appear peaceful, relaxed, and glowing as if radiating a sense of happiness and strength, as well as exhibiting a heightened state of awareness. When the moment of death approaches, individuals experience certain sensations which reflect imminent departure. Many, at this point are overtaken by fear and despair.

2) Restoration Stage

The restoration stage, or moment of death, refers to the soul's returning of the physical body to the primal pool of material, or atomic substance; the etheric body to the primordial ethers; and the prana to the universal reservoir of life energy. This process is followed by the soul's return to its natural environment of spiritual energy, abandoning the physical plane of existence and the vehicles utilized for the present incarnation.

Overview of External and Internal Changes at the Moment of Death

Dying, the individuals may instinctively try to hold on to physical life, although they would often feel perturbed when attempts are made by medical personnel to bring them forcibly back or to maintain life, however well meaning such efforts may be. In cases when death occurs over long time, the soul alternates between exiting and reentering the physical body, although there is an instant when a firm decision is made by the soul to separate from the physical body. At the moment of death, the acceptance of the fact that the physical body is a dense, gross, trapping vehicle becomes easier now.

Due to a strong desire to communicate with loved ones, the form of dying individuals may appear to relatives and other persons close to them through a mechanism of mental projection of the personality, or direct projection of the astral body. Such a mental projection happens as a thought transmission, which imprints the consciousness of the contacted individual with the image of the dying one. In this way, dying individuals can project their forms either as mental images or as the actual astral bodies, to other rooms, or even to distant places.

The physical senses progressively fade, thus sight, touch, and movement become obtuse, with the sense of hearing being the last to go. The limbs feel sluggish and heavy, with sensations that progress to the entire physical body in unison with a vague feeling of collapsing. Then the physical body grows numb, and the identity of the body disappears. As the physical senses fade away, the psychic senses become sharper and the dying person may experience clairvoyant and clairaudient phenomena, being able to see and hear what is happening in other places.

Individuals passing through the door of death might also experience telepathic phenomena, able to communicate with distant loved ones, either living or dead. Since the concepts of time and space, as we know them, are disappearing as well, it is not uncommon for dying people to feel the proximity of those closest to them, regardless of whether they are present, as such closeness is felt in the heart. Nonetheless, dying individuals generally regard the physical presence of others at the scene as very comforting, especially if those are close to them.

Following the will of the soul, the etheric body of the individual prepares for extrication from its physical counterpart. Internally, the person will hear sounds, resulting from the process of disengaging that may be similar to those made by breaking ice, the banging of metal, electronic beeps, loud ringing, explosions, buzzing, rushing wind, or running water. Later in the process other kind of sounds may be heard, such as bells, choirs, or musical instruments like flutes, trumpets, or drums.

Breathing becomes extremely shallow and slow. There are sensations like tingling, alternating feelings of cold and heat, increasing pressure followed by lightness, and finally a sense of floating then spinning. Strong, and rapid vibrations, which increase in intensity, lead to a feeling of being absorbed by something. There is no pain then, only calmness and silence.

Just before completely exiting the physical body, the soul experiences the first encounter with the Light and the first life review.

Next, the part of the silver cord, or magnetic energy thread, linking the etheric body to the physical body is partially severed, and the individuals have the sensation of moving out of the body at a high speed through a long, dark tunnel. Then the soul comes to the second encounter with the Light and the second life review. The soul departs carrying within itself all pertinent information about the individual, which is contained in "chips" of etheric substance and prana - the permanent physical, astral, and mental atoms, constituting the so-called memory of the soul.

Then the minimal portion of the silver cord still remaining is totally severed, and the soul is completely free from the physical body. After its exit, the soul undergoes some episodes still related to the physical dimension of its previous life. Soon thereafter the etheric body is likewise released by the soul and stays for a while around the abandoned physical body. The entire departure of the soul may take from a few minutes to as long as approximately thirty six hours.

Very sensitive people present at the time of someone's death may perceive a scent left by the exiting soul, which can range from one similar to the smell of incense or flowers to a fetid odor, depending on the level of spiritual development achieved by the dying persons. Such sensitive people may also see a delicate gleam or a flash of light coming from the body of dying individuals when the soul departs, while others might experience a sense of rejoicing.

In fact, if we could expand our perceptual faculties, we would discover that Nature generally responds to the important human passages of life. In the case of death, Nature frequently sends messages that may take the form of warnings prior to death and the form of something which brings consolation following death. Nature can also send messages in the form of sounds of animals, strange behavior of birds, unusual weather manifestations, shooting stars, or items braking and clocks stopping.

When the soul has departed from the physical vehicle and the silver cord has been totally severed, the etheric body is still interpenetrated by the energies of the subtle bodies and the soul, appearing as a diffuse contour of the former physical body and comprising the energy of the thought forms dead people have about themselves throughout their lives. At this point, some attraction between the etheric body and its former physical vehicle still exists, causing the individual to remain near the dead body for a while.

Immediately after departing from the physical body and while still inhabiting the etheric body, the soul finds itself in a semi-consciousness, dream-like state but peaceful, unless great emotional disturbance is occurring around the dead physical body. In many occasions, persons in the house or nearby environment visually perceive this etheric double as a vague silhouette or shiny mist that is silent, immobile, and nonresponsive, although they may appear with a fixed expression reflecting some emotion or thought of the deceased, such as terror, sorrow, or confusion. This situation may result from extreme anxiety at the moment of death, powerful thoughts focused on someone left behind, unfinished business of the dying, or external turmoil around the dying person. Next, the etheric body is left totally empty by the soul. Such etheric shells, which can be seen by people who possess astral vision, for example in graveyards, are what we call ghosts.

The recently abandoned physical body begins to deteriorate. Its particles, which had been held together as a whole organism by the force of prana circulating through the etheric body and directed by the soul, now scatter.

The etheric body also slowly disintegrates, releasing its prana, which is then returned to the universal pool of energy related to the etheric body of the planet Earth. The dissolution of the etheric body is aided if the physical body is cremated, since the strong attraction exerted by matter and form is thus eliminated. The vanishing of the etheric body may occur in a time span of four hours to over sixty days. Meanwhile, the etheric vehicle remains in close proximity to the physical body. If the dead person happens to be undeveloped, it might take a long time for the etheric body to disappear, and it might linger close to its physical counterpart due to strong material attraction. Conversely, if the dead individual is more advanced, the etheric body can disappear quickly. Thus, for the physical and etheric bodies death can be understood as the dissolution and transformation of the form that constituted a whole organism.

The restoration stage along the process of death is then completed with the atomic substance of the physical body and the energy of the etheric body having been restored to their original sources and the soul — donning the garments of emotions and lower mind having moved to some level of the astral plane of existence.

After the soul gives the signal for death, instantly the internal physiological processes begin. The glands of the endocrine system produce a substance which, running through the blood stream, triggers a reflex from the brain, where the consciousness thread is anchored, and then affect the heart, where the life thread is anchored, leading to a comatose condition or loss of consciousness.

Next a very potent vibration coursing through the etheric body causes looseness in the nadis (channels of energy), beginning at the level of the eyes, detaching the nadis from the corresponding branches of the nervous system. Eventually this leads to the separation of the etheric body from its physical counterpart. However, at first, the etheric body still interpenetrates every part of the physical body. The loosening of the nadis represents the first sign of the desire to yield the physical body. While this happens, the person usually remains relaxed, fearless, and peaceful. At this stage, commonly there is a pause in the process.

After loosening its tight association with the physical nervous system, the etheric body begins to gradually detach from the extremities of the body and to collect itself at the level of the chakra that will serve as the door for its exit from the physical body. The soul still abides within the physical body, in the main central channel of energy (Sushumna). Here the first encounter with the Light occurs, as well as the first life review. The Light often appears as a luminous darkness, sometimes with a violet tint and represents the naked, true nature of the mind. If the person realizes it is a reflection of the self and is able to merge with it, enlightenment and liberation become a possibility. The first life review occurs in the form of a rapid projection of images showing the entire life of the dying person in sequence or with the totality of images flashing simultaneously. This is originated by photon particles moving at the speed of light as the contents of the energy centers, or chakras, are being released. The person objectively looks at himself/herself, comprehending the purpose of his/her life and the foremost inclination of that life, as a whole, is profoundly imprinted into the soul. This review, in a way, is more physical and matter of fact.

Up to then, the etheric body has been prepared for withdrawal, the physical body is disengaged and already answering to the calling of the spirit of the Earth, while the soul turns its attention inwardly and focuses on the astral and mental vehicles.

The process of the soul leaving the physical body can be better distinguished by those who die naturally from old age than by those dying from disease or suddenly due to an accident. Spiritually advanced individuals have total awareness of this occurrence.

At this time, usually a second brief pause takes place. This is a crucial juncture in the process, since it is when physical life could be resumed by the individual if the soul decides to do so for whatever reason. If this happens, the etheric body again expands and interpenetrates the physical body, allowing the elemental of the physical body to take charge of it once more. At this particular point the only contact remaining between the physical and etheric bodies is at the level of either the Solar Plexus chakra or the Heart chakra or some of the centers in the head. In addition, contact continues to exist through two minor chakras located in the area of the lungs, the last of the energy centers to dissolve within the etheric substance, as well as the two energy centers that will be first reactivated by the soul when physical life is to be restored.

If the person is still strongly desirous of perpetuating physical existence, a desperate struggle occurs between the physical elemental force and the will of the soul, slowing the natural course of the process of death. However, if the soul is still focused on leaving definitely the physical vehicle, at this point departs taking with it the subtle energy bodies. To make this possible, part of the silver cord is broken and the soul, donning ventures of light, exits the physical body through one of the portals, depending on circumstances of dying individuals: The Solar Plexus chakra, a common tendency for infants and adults who have lived a life primarily focused on the physical and emotional levels; The Heart chakra, which is the case for moderately developed persons who are benevolent and caring; or The Head chakras (Throat, Third Eye, and Crown), which is the case for very advanced individuals. The chakras are sealed with dense woven strands of etheric energy that must be punctured at the moment of exit.

The overall inclination and the main focus of the physical life of dying individuals have an important influence on the manner and place of the soul's exit from the physical body at the moment of death, just as this influence the rest of the process.

Ideally, spiritual work enabling individuals to govern the emotional natures and focus on the mental and spiritual worlds, should prepare them for the soul's departure from the physical body at the highest level possible (fifth, sixth, or, better seventh chakra) since such an occurrence would present the best possibility for enlightenment.

The soul, now enshrouded with the mental, emotional, and etheric bodies, exits the physical body and the remaining minimal part of the silver cord is severed, terminating all contact with the physical vehicle.

Overview of Changes in the Energy Centers, or Chakras, at the Moment of Death (The dissolution of the elements)
The flying soul of the dying person focuses consciousness on each energy center, or chakra, while traveling upward through the three main central energy channels (Sushumna, Ida, and Pingala) prior to its final departure. The individual witnesses the successive dissolution of the internal elements at each chakra level, sensing various physical, visual, and audio phenomena linked specifically to each one of these stages.

When a person is dying, the internal elements start to fade one into the other, first the grosser or dense forms followed by the subtler ones. As this occurs, the bio-field of etheric substance and energy, or etheric body, simultaneously breaks its connections with the physical body.

Thus, the inner element earth, which correlates with the first energy center, or Root chakra evanesces into the subtler inner element water, which belongs to the second energy center or Sacral chakra. This, in turn, transmutes into the inner element fire (chemical heat and light), which corresponds to the third energy center, or Solar Plexus chakra. Subsequently, fire dissolves into the inner element air, which pertains to the fourth energy center, or Heart chakra, and this finally transmute to the inner element ether, related to the fifth energy center, or Throat chakra. Ether then shifts into pure, expansive and limitless consciousness.

Each transmutation of the inner elements is accompanied by particular internal visions and sensations resulting from projections revealing different scenes, colors, lights, and sounds, arising at the level of each chakra as their energetic contents are released. So at this stage of the process of death the individual faces a variety of audio and visual phenomena, which are both experienced subjectively and objectively. These projections actually originate within ourselves and reflect what is in our minds at all levels, from the subconscious to the super-conscious. Ideally they should be viewed as if we were watching a movie, recognizing and accepting them as the products of our own minds. If we can do this, we can merge with them without shock or fear.

It is not desirable to become entrapped at any of these levels by engaging with these phenomena and then reacting to them with fear, because this would produce an instant constriction of the electromagnetic field with the consequence that the individual experiences only a grayish, dull state, finding it impossible to think or see anything. The prayers and loving thoughts of living individuals left behind can significantly help dying people to avoid this pit fall.

Chakra Stages
First Stage: Root Chakra
This stage is marked by the internal element of earth being absorbed by the internal element of water. The physical sensation is feeling cold and exceedingly weak, like fading away. The sense of vision declines and everything turns cloudy and ambiguous, like a view of things under running water. The predominant color is yellow, and the inner visual scenes are of destruction by earthquakes and inundation.

Second Stage: Sacral Chakra
This stage is marked by the internal element of water dissolving in the internal element of fire. The physical sensation is a feeling of heat, drying out and being extremely thirsty as the body fluids evaporate. The sense of touch deteriorates, and the individual becomes numb. Attachment begins to disappear. The main color is white, and the inner visual scenes are smoky scenarios of flooding with the person being submerged in smoke.

Third Stage: Solar Plexus Chakra
This stage is marked by the internal element of fire dissipating within the inner element of air. The sensation is of extreme heat and then cold, as body heat is lost. The sense of smell, as well as the energy of desire, disappears. The predominant color is red, and the inner visual scenes are of everything in flames and the individual surrounded by infinity of sparks that look like fireflies.

Fourth Stage: Heart chakra

This stage is marked by the internal element of air vanishing into the internal element of ether and the consequence is that all volitional functions and breathing cease. The sense of taste disappears and the energy of competition fades away. The predominant color is green, and the inner visual scenes are of powerful winds blowing. The electromagnetic field breaks up. Individuals hear with their inner ears a roaring that sounds like gigantic masses of ice breaking apart and experience themselves as encircled by a single flame. At this point, clinical death is declared. The first encounter with the Light occurs when the internal elements have already dissolved.

These stages of dissolution of the internal elements may be experienced by individuals in varying degrees, from the mildest forms to the most intense, depending on the person's involvement and focus of attention. Generally, individuals have an inclination to recoil from these phenomena, due to either shock or fear, especially if they are unprepared. Or, they may even become unconscious. The majority of people go through these stages without being able to recognize them and without knowing what is happening to them, thus they are unable to take advantage of the opportunities these stages offer for experiencing freedom, bliss, or some level of enlightenment.

To experience these stages in the best possible manner, it is important to do the following:

— Maintain the understanding that all these phenomena are only projections of the mind, that they are not external events.
— Remain only a witness, without either recoiling from, becoming engaged with, or reacting to the phenomena with fear.
— Try to help the soul's exit by focusing on breathing up, level after level.
— Remain awake and alert while experiencing the phenomena, avoiding the tendency to recoil.
— Invoke the help of a spiritual master or teacher.
— Have a support person assisting with voice commands and gentle touch.

Stages beyond the Dissolution of the Inner Elements

Fifth Stage: Gross Consciousness to Luminance

This is the stage that advances the individual from a condition of gross consciousness (internal element of ether) to a state of luminance. During this stage, the "yang", or masculine energy flowing through the channel Pingala is emptied into the main central channel Sushumna. This energy current descends from the brain area to the heart. The individual experiences being surrounded by an infinite sky bathed in silvery moonlight.

Sixth Stage: Luminance to Radiance

At this stage, the "yin", or femimine energy that courses through the channel Ida is emptied into the central channel Sushumna in an ascending movement from the Root chakra toward the heart area. The individual has the experience of being surrounded by a vast orange sunlit sky.

Seventh Stage: Radiance to Imminence

At this stage, the individual becomes an entity existing in subtle consciousness or in the abstract mind. The "yang" and "yin" energies merge at the Heart chakra, enveloping the soul. The dying person is aware of being surrounded by an immense sky of bright, purplish darkness and feels engulfed by a quiescent emptiness.

Eight Stage: Imminence to Translucency

During this stage the individual progresses into a realm of clear light. This is the first encounter with the Light and provides an important opportunity for enlightenment, if the person recognizes it as a reflection of the self and as the Original Reality, perfectly unbound and formless, perfectly peaceful and blissful. The crisscrossed energies of the left and right central channels (Ida and Pingala) around the heart suddenly disentangle, leaving the soul free to exit the physical body. The individual's consciousness is beyond duality. This could be considered the real moment of death.

Now, a tunnel between different dimensions opens in front of the departing soul, and a bright, white light becomes visible beyond it. The person acquires awareness of another reality and feels pulled into it. At first the sensation is that of floating, then of increasingly rapid movement through space, feeling like a rock projected at a high velocity. Then the individual may lose consciousness; hear the sound of humming or of a melodious flute, and sense a confluence of energies at heart level, a feeling that typifies the encounter with a larger force, or cosmic energy.

Meanwhile, the disclosure of different aspects of the mind continues with releasing energy taking the shape of visions, sounds, and lights, which destroy the lower ego — if the person can transcend duality by recognizing them not as external phenomena but as parts of the self — presenting an opportunity for liberation through experiencing wholeness and non duality. If the individuals miss this opportunity, they may feel overwhelmed and terrified by the energies coming out of their own mind and may become aware of; and instinctively attracted to dimmer lights associated with different realms of physical existence, reflecting the predominant negative emotions and customary tendencies of the ego, which can lead to the specific conditions of a new incarnation later. Also the departed individual may see others nearby, likely already deceased relatives and friends.

In essence, what happens after clinical death and the exit of the soul is like a re-tracing of different levels of the mind from the personal conscious, to the personal subconscious, to the psychic, to the collective subconscious, and to the super conscious.

During the progression of the soul through the tunnel, an ideal situation can be created by trying to remain at the center of it and aim for the brightest light, which is perceived at the end of the tunnel, representing the second encounter with the Light and another chance for enlightenment. The magnificent white Light is so brilliant that it could provoke extreme fear in the persons, causing them to instinctively recoil from it. However, if the dying individual is knowledgeable about the death experience, is guided by a support person, is free from fear, remembers to focus consciousness on a spiritual teacher and can identify the Light as a reflection of the self, once again enlightenment may be possible.

Between the two extreme situations of either recoiling from the Light or becoming unified with it, the individual may experience various degrees of proximity with the splendorous Light, which is always welcoming, radiates love, wisdom, calmness, and supreme understanding so that the individual feels profoundly invigorated. The Light might appear as a figure of light or simply as pure energy of light, but it is always experienced by the dying person as a powerful Being who communicates telepathically and it is nothing other than our own Higher Self or Monadic Self. After the Light transmits a sense of love and peace, the individual is then compelled to examine the recent life. This is the second life review, which occurs as a rapid visual projection of the earthly life either in its entirety or only its most important moments. This review is not only visual but also emotional since the dead persons can feel not only their own feelings but also the feelings of all others with whom they interacted in that life period. As well, individuals can clearly see how their thoughts, intentions, and actions affected others and circumstances, revealing how they did or did not benefit the entire world. The dead person is aware of the lessons learned and those that remain to be learned.

The only judgment about the individual's life is made by the person's soul, which instantly assesses with perfect justice, in accord with its highest level of consciousness. In addition, the dead person feels profoundly grateful for the opportunity of life on Earth. Thus we see that once the soul exits the physical and etheric bodies goes through imminent experiences that still incriminate the physical dimension of existence.

After the second encounter with the Light, there are successive meetings with various lights representing different dimensions of consciousness and providing additional opportunities for the individual to merge with them. Thus, during the process of death, especially at the early stages, dying individuals have several chances to choose between liberation from the cycle of reincarnation or returning again to the world of duality, ignorance, and past habits.

The individual's soul, enshrouded with emotional and mental vestures, is momentarily free from its encasement in a physical body and now exists at some level of the astral plane. The dead persons soon realize that individuality is not lost, that their real self still endures and has been unaffected by physical death, although the true character of the person cannot be concealed in any way.

Often the individual rejoins friends and relatives who have already gone through the transition of death, as well spirit guides. All these beings are seen as spheres of light with different colors, and they may transmit messages. Communication is telepathic, and questions receive answers instantly. In addition, intense bonds of love are easily felt.

The astral body is perceived by the individual in the following diverse ways:

- As formless and translucent

- As a vaporous sphere
- As an oval egg
- As a pear-shaped body
- As an ambiguous contour of a human body, with extremities and a head
- As an outline of the former physical body

The individuals are in a freer state, looking at their former physical and etheric bodies, often first in a dreamlike state of consternation and dismay, then later, with more vibrant and clear perceptions. The mind is hyper lucid, vision and hearing are acute and vivid. The persons are totally cognizant of what is happening in the physical world around them, able to witness everything as invisible observers. In many cases, when the individual has developed the capacity to be fully awake, communications with the living left behind are possible during the first weeks or months after death. These contacts could occur in a direct manner or as signs or happenings that convey to the receiver some aspect of the personality of the departed one.

Characteristics of the Moment of Death under Specific Circumstances
Unexpected, Abrupt and Violent Death by Accident or Murder
In these cases, the separation of the soul from the physical and etheric bodies does not happen in a slow, step-by-step manner but precociously and hastily, with the consequence that the soul retains some material elements from the physical and etheric bodies since there is an incomplete dissolution of the internal elements, although such retention is only temporary. This circumstance makes it easier for the soul to appear in a visual form to the persons who remain alive on Earth or to perform some acts that involve physical force. The moment of death of these individuals also includes the first encounter with the Light, the first life review, the tunnel experience, the second encounter with the Light, and the second life review, although these events happen very rapidly. The individual is pretty much awake and alert immediately after death but very confused and may remain involved in the situation we call earthbound.

Suicide Death
If the individual commits suicide, physical life is destroyed prematurely and opportunities for spiritual growth are denied to the soul. Consequently, the electromagnetic bonds with the physical body and hence with the physical

dimension remain strong until what would have normally been the due time of death for that person. Such individuals experience a sensation of being extremely heavy and dense. They undergo the first encounter with the Light and first life review, the tunnel experience, and the second encounter with the Light and second life review, all in extremely rapid succession. They become aware of the significance of their act and how meaningful their lives could have been for them had they chosen to remain alive. Such persons will almost immediately experience the condition known as the slumber of the soul, suffer unimaginable torments in a restless, feverish dream state, and remain earthbound but unable to communicate with anybody. In such cases, the soul is not liberated and remains linked to the same individuals or conditions that the dead person tried to avoid by committing suicide.

Capital Punishment Death

When individuals are put to death prematurely as a result of capital punishment, the soul experiences similar conditions as for other cases when the soul is forced out of the physical body. The difference lies in the disposition of the so-called criminal whose life is ended. After the individual's death they find themselves in an earthbound state of fear, anger and hatred. Such souls tend to associate with like ones and wander through the lower astral worlds looking for situations in which they can have an influence on humans of weaker minds, inducing them to kill or hurt others. Thus, all that capital punishment does is to remove the possibilities for those individuals to correct their behavior, be rehabilitated, and experience spiritual growth. Therefore, capital punishment is not the correct solution for improving our societies. It should be part of the spiritual duty of any society to give such disturbed and undeveloped beings assistance.

In all of these situations of sudden death, either by accident, murder, suicide, or capital punishment, it is of special importance to cremate the physical body since its quick dissolution lessens the material pull exerted on the soul that makes it remain in an earthbound state and it may even help the soul realize its new condition and do something to obtain some sort of help.

Death of a Spiritual Master

Spiritual masters are individuals who have direct contact with their Higher Selves, or Monads. The Monad and not the soul directs the individuality in its periods of reincarnation. Spiritual masters bring about physical death intentionally, in accordance with a plan and with full consciousness clearly knowing that a cycle of planetary life has ended for them. Thus the physical body is abandoned peacefully and gracefully.

CHAPTER III

Stages of the Process of Death
The Intermission:
Stage 3 - Shedding Stage
Stage 4 - Assimilation Stage

3) Shedding Stage

The intermission refers to the span of life of the individual soul in the astral and mental planes of existence, after physical death has occurred and prior to reincarnation and the next period of physical life on Earth.

The shedding stage in the process of death, which begins the intermission period, is the soul's gradual disengagement from the emotional and lower mental bodies, occurring at different levels of the astral and mental planes. Generally this stage comprises the following:

— Invigoration of the soul
— First slumber of the soul
— Meeting with the Karmic Council and Reorientation
— Life of the soul in the astral plane
— Second death and second slumber of the soul (passing from the astral to the mental plane and leaving behind the emotional body)
— Life of the soul in the lower regions of the mental plane (leaving behind the lower mental body)

Once the soul has disengaged from the physical and etheric bodies, it undergoes certain experiences which still encompass the physical dimension. At
this point, the partially liberated soul is able to see and hear the individuals
left behind in the physical plane. Sensing their grief, the soul may fall prey
to despair, which makes its departure more difficult.

After physical death and posterior to the initial encounters with the
Light, there occur subtle perceptions of lights of diverse colors, rays, and
sounds, which represent new chances for attaining different degrees of enlightenment if they are recognized as such by the individual. These occurrences mark the soul's arrival to the dreamlike world of the astral plane, and
the beginning of intermission. The individual understands that existence has
not ended, and all the faculties and habits of the mind are still intact, including memory, thinking, questioning, and reasoning. As well, feeling, seeing,
hearing, and moving remain, but at this point are qualities of the astral body
in which the individual is now functioning.

Under these new conditions, the soul has heightened perceptivity, which
results in the manifestation of visions and sounds of a disconcerting magnitude. Facing these experiences, the individual often panics. In addition, in
the midst of this circumstance, the contents of the person's instinctive subconscious mind can automatically and rapidly surface, causing extreme reactions in the individual — either of joy or terror. All the incidents and
images appearing are determined by the contents of our own minds. If we
have been influenced by fear of suffering and damage, our tendency will be
to react with terror, and this state, in turn, can produce even more disturbing
occurrences. If we succumb to this panic state, our energy field automatically
contracts, we guard ourselves increasingly, and we descend into vicious cir-
cles of negativity. Therefore, it is fundamentally important not to give in to
fear but instead to stay fearless and calm.

While a person is experiencing life within a physical body, the emotional or astral body is constituted by astral substance from the seven
subdivisions of the astral plane, which are mixed together. However, after
physical death and once away from the physical body the astral body undergoes a transformation in its appearance, preparing it to go through
several stages of purification and gradual disintegration, a necessary
process for a more complete liberation of the soul. The transformation
of the astral body consists of a rearrangement of the particles of astral
substance belonging to the various subdivisions of the astral plane so that

they form seven concentric layers separated by their vibratory rate and density, the densest being the outer band, and the subtlest being the innermost band.

The individual is confined, for the moment, to the astral region, which corresponds to the outer layer of their astral or emotional body. From the former description, we can infer how important it is to conscientiously work, during physical life, toward the purification of our emotional selves.

During physical life, our focus is primarily on how to function in the material plane through a physical body. But after physical death, this focus is, of necessity, shifted. One of the first tasks awaiting us during the intermission is to refocus consciousness toward the spiritual worlds and awareness of the new faculties we now possess. It is extremely beneficial if we, after death, could acknowledge the stages of life in the astral plane as a process of letting go of those bodies that are no longer needed — physical, etheric, and emotional. During our stay in the astral plane, our awareness continues to increase like the gradual growth we undergo during physical life.

Invigoration of the Soul

Souls, upon reentering the spirit world after physical death exhibit different degrees of exhaustion, damage, and contamination from the recent life, therefore their energy needs to be restituted with the help of spirit guides and, many times, with the help of soul group mates. Souls with damaged energy are given infusions of powerful energy from their spirit guides. Also, gaps in the auric field of these individuals are sealed and their disrupted energy is rearranged to make it whole.

Souls that are more evolved often return to the spirit world undamaged and do not need this help, while individuals that have lived physical lives repeatedly and deliberately performing acts of cruelty and harming others, return to the spirit world as severely damaged souls requiring more intense modalities of treatment for recovery.

Thereafter, these souls are taken to places where they can be in isolation and the process of recovery continues with treatment by spirit guides and other specialized spirit beings. The cleansing and strengthening of these souls' energies is done by further reshaping of energy, infusion of pure white light, and the use of sound and color vibrations.

First Slumber of the Soul

Following the second life review—the revelation of the subconscious layers of memory, secondary encounters with lights, and invigoration procedures the individual falls temporarily asleep. This slumber of the soul is necessary for individuals to become familiar with the new circumstances and existence in this environment. In this condition, the soul inhabits its astral body, which is carefully safeguarded so nothing can harm it. This situation may be compared to that of a baby growing in a mother's womb, preparing to be born in a new world, in this case into the astral world.

The sleeping of the soul may be shorter or longer for different people. This interval provides the ideal situation for the individual to be able to transfer the focus of consciousness from one world to the other and also it can be considered as the third life review. The soul brings with it a condensed chronicle of the recent life, encompassing all likes, dislikes, desires, and goals.

During the entire period of the soul's slumber, the dead person is still influenced by stimuli from the physical plane of Earth. While slumbering, the soul elects either to cling to the physical plane of existence or release attachments to it. If the latter is not done, the soul undergoes dreamlike experiences which disturb its peaceful sleep and are initiated by different emotions such as fear, strong desires, or love.

Individuals who have experienced a natural death and have been at peace during the moment of death, enter into the slumber state soon and without difficulties. They are not usually disturbed by dreamlike conditions and can rest peacefully through this phase, progressing effortlessly to the next stage. Nonetheless, there are two situations which may give rise to dreams of the slumbering soul:

One situation is when the dying individuals entertain in their mind potent desires and emotions connected to the Earth life, for instance, feeling regret, guilt, hate, or frustration because of unfinished business, or preoccupation with people left behind. The other situation is when an individual still alive have intense thoughts, emotions, and desires relating to the dying person, often arising from feelings of love. In both circumstances, the intense vibrations produced by these passionate feelings may trigger like vibrations in the astral, or emotional body of the discarnate individual, thus disturbing the soul's slumber, resulting in one of the following conditions: an agitated, delirious state with dreamlike experiences and non volitional attempts at communication with the living ones through a kind of telepathy; some degree of awakening, although it may be compared to the condition we call som-nambulism during physical life; or a complete arousal from the slumber, recollection of the recent life and a strong desire to return to the loved ones on Earth. This kind of disturbance of the resting soul produces deep torment, since the individual is pulled by earthly ties and the natural evolution of the soul is thus hindered. However, the time comes when such souls grow exhausted and ultimately fall into deep sleep.

A different situation occurs in cases of abrupt death, either by accident, disease, or murder. The souls of such individuals do not fall immediately asleep but remain awake, with their mental faculties functioning, aware of the events on Earth life — to the point of not realizing that they have died — and experiencing emotions such as bewilderment, frustration, and unhappiness. However, in due time they finally fall into sleep, after receiving advice from astral guides.

The time souls remain slumbering varies for different people. During this stage, the soul's growth continues, and it does not awake until the maximum degree of integration of experiences and evolution for that particular soul has occurred and the person is fully prepared to face the challenges of the new existence in their corresponding astral sub-plane.

Individuals who are not very developed spend a shorter time in this state, while those who are more developed need a longer time in this state since they are more prepared to reject the negative aspects of their emotional/mental makeup and thus have a greater potential for achieving a higher level of purification and integration.

At some point, the individual soul regains consciousness, rapidly releasing the lower components of its nature in accordance with the individual's level of evolution, and gaining a new awareness about existence on the astral plane. Each soul is fated to inhabit the astral sub-plane that correlates with the outer layer of its astral body. Later on, after the gradual dissolution of remnants of lower nature, the soul attains the sub-plane which vibrates in unison with its most elevated aspects.

Meeting with the Karmic Council and Reorientation

After the conclusion of a life period, individuals appear before the Karmic Council on which occasion the results of their recent life are presented to the seven Lords of Karma in a completely neutral manner. This can be considered as a fourth life review, which reveals the degree to which the person's consciousness has evolved and how much the individual has contributed to the collective development of humanity. The extent of spiritual evolvement of a person can be clearly realized by observing their causal body. Nevertheless, this review is not limited only to the immediate past life but covers the progress of the soul trough all other past lives.

The seven Lords of Karma who constitute the Karmic Council are spiritually advanced beings and Ascended Masters whose function is to aid evolving human beings in balancing negative and positive karmic debts, transforming into pure divine light, and finally ascending to higher spiritual levels on the way back Home. These wise spiritual beings exhibit immense compassion and patience, having a welcoming, encouraging and loving but firm attitude toward the souls being evaluated.

Every soul transits through the Hall of Karma in the etheric realm of our planet and appears before the Karmic Council, both after exiting the physical body at death and again prior to reincarnation on Earth.

The great majority of individual souls experience slumbers before appearing to the Karmic Council, and has already had opportunities to review their recent life and judge it for themselves from the perspective of the chances offered to them during that life to help with their spiritual advancement. Those who are extremely advanced in their spiritual evolution may skip the slumber period and quickly appear before the Karmic Council by themselves. In addition there are souls who never appear before the Karmic Council due to special conditions of their deaths, such as suicide and capital punishment. Such individuals are usually not prepared to appear before the Lords of Karma because of the traumatic characteristics of their deaths, and so their souls need a prolonged period of slumber and rehabilitation.

The individuals, who are more spiritually advanced, as well as those who are average but have shown some spiritual interest during earth life, appear before the Karmic Council fully conscious and accompanied by their spirit guides. But the majority of people make their appearance to the Karmic Council in a semi-conscious state, in groups, and under the supervision of spirit guardians.

As summaries of people's recent lives are presented to the Karmic Council, its members listen impartially. Their mission is not to judge or punish but to aid individuals to grow spiritually in the most favorable manner and plan better for future experiences, always respecting the Law of Karma, or Law of Cause and Effect. They are in charge of determining the portion of karmic debt that each person must balance during a given lifetime, among the sum total of karma amassed by the persons during their different lives on Earth. The remaining karmic debt endures quiescent in the etheric realms waiting to be neutralized during succeeding life periods. Thus they help individuals to make amends when needed and direct souls to the best environment for their spiritual progress. An additional function of the Karmic Council is organizing the reincarnation of souls in earthly physical bodies, since there are too many souls transiting through this line of planetary evolution by attending Earth school and only one third of them can be given the chance of experiencing planetary life at a given time. Moreover members of the Karmic Council are concerned with guiding souls to reincarnate surrounded by the best possible conditions for each one's spiritual growth.

Awaken souls are cognizant of their mistakes and understand perfectly the consequences of their actions while incarnated, mainly if they harmed others during their physical lives. The purpose of Karmic Council meetings is to evaluate and review the behavior and actions of souls during incarnation, considering especially the following:

— Major choices of souls.
— Accountability for their actions.
— How they used power.
— How they demonstrated love.
— Opinion of the individuals about how they feel the physical vehicle helped or delayed their evolution.
— How the individual souls interacted with the physical brains.
— Up to what degree the inner essence of the souls maintained integrity in terms of values and aspirations. In other words, what was the level of contamination and damage to the souls by interfacing with matter.
— How the individuals feel about having another reincarnation.

Soon after appearing before the Karmic Council, the more advanced souls begin resolving their karmic debts and attend exclusive schools where they receive guidance by spiritual teachers. Less developed souls are directed to their corresponding sub-planes of the astral world, where they are instructed on the purpose of their existence and their lives on Earth, as well as they receive orientation about the astral life.

The souls who appear before the Karmic Council in groups and in a semiconscious state are directed, and accompanied by spiritual guardians, to appropriate astral sub-planes, where they are helped to awaken, even if only minimally.

The souls who have lead predominantly disharmonious, or criminal lives on Earth endure some kind of suffering as the consequence of their actions, which is not a punishment but a corrective measure that results from the working of the Law of Karma.

Further, individuals who during Earth life exhibited extreme selfishness, using any means to pursue material gain, who had an addiction problem; and those who perversely enjoyed the pain of others are detained in a sub-plane very near to the Earth existence, tied by their self-created magnetic strings in an earthbound condition.

Another group of souls, those who did not believe in life after death, may be guided to return to the region of the soul's slumber to further rest and get better prepared for life in the astral realm.

In summary, souls are spiritually assessed by the Karmic Council and thereafter directed to the appropriate sub-plane of the astral realm where they continue expanding in comprehension and growth under the teaching and guidance of celestial beings. This is an orientation period with our spirit guides and it takes place before souls reunite with their corresponding soul groups.

Individuals who terminated their lives intentionally (suicide), as I mention before, do not appear before the Karmic Council and are offered, by their spirit guides, some possibilities for help and healing. First of all they are shown various choices they could have made other than suicide and they are allowed to experience a different outcome, with the purpose of broadening their understanding.

The possibilities for them range from being subjected to intense regeneration of their energy, the option of quickly returning to a new incarnation in order to recover lost time (usually this is the option for individuals who committed suicide for the first time), the option of isolation in natural environments without contact with other beings (this is the case of individuals who have committed suicide repeatedly), to the option of continuing reincarnating in another planetary world, since many individuals never adjust to planet Earth.

Suicide is never a possibility included in a life plan as a way of balancing karma. It is never a prearranged option for anybody.

Life of the Soul in the Astral Realm

After death, souls first appear on the astral plane. Each plane of existence encompasses innumerable sub-planes which are characterized by different vibration rates and are populated by souls of like frequencies. In the case of the astral plane, where our first steps after physical death take place, there are lower, intermediate, and higher sub-planes. The mental state of individuals here consists of the total sum of growth achieved up to that point during Earth life, through practicing tolerance, moderation, compassion, understanding, and love.

The person still experiences living in a body, which now is the emotional, or astral body. Usually this body assumes the form of the individual's self-image during their recent life on Earth. At first it is the self-image they had at the time of death or the last time they felt good, while later it is the self-image they had when they felt the happiest in their recent life. Still later it may not resemble so closely the person's self-image of the earthly life.

The person's astral body is psycho-plastic, as well as the surrounding environment. It can easily metamorphose depending on how the individual feels, perceives, thinks, and interacts with others. But nothing can be hidden, and their true self is clearly exposed.

The environment of the astral plane results solely from the thought forms of the souls in it. Thus the sceneries of the sub-planes depict the amalgamated blend of the mental images of its inhabitants. Souls have several possibilities on the astral plane: to spontaneously create their environment, to visit other already existing settings, or to add their own creations to an existing environment. Those souls possessing a similar set of mental images reside together in a given sub-plane, influencing the general qualities of the realm. So we are able to bring about consciously our own environment on the astral plane, which is contrary to what happens on Earth, where the environment greatly affects and influences us.

The astral sub-planes correlate with levels of consciousness of the individuals who have lived a physical life on Earth and encompass all those conditions that humans designate as purgatory, hell, and heaven, as well as intermediate states. These conditions are transitory, originate in the minds of individuals, and are the result of actions initiated during life on Earth. If we think in a positive way, have faith, meditate, pray, and offer our light, we live in "heaven." On the other hand, if we think in a negative way, judge, and criticize others, we live in "hell."

The purpose of these conditions, including those involving suffering, is to facilitate further purification and learning. Such conditions reflect the teaching device known as the Law of Karma.

Time and space as we know them do not exist on the astral plane, since there is not a physical brain that registers time in a linear fashion according to a sequence of episodes. There are no space barriers, thus moving is easy and rapid. Astral traveling occurs by shifting from one degree of vibration to another, guided by the imagination and feelings about places or persons we desire to encounter.

The substance of the astral plane is subtler and more malleable than that of the physical plane, and its vibrations are faster in general; however, within the astral plane we encounter a variation of vibration rates which constitute the different sub-planes. Therefore, we encounter varied conditions of existence in the astral realm, which is inhabited by souls who conform to the vibratory characteristics of each sub-plane. Due to the principle of attraction, within the Law of Vibration, individuals are naturally drawn toward the specific condition for which they are suited.

The lower sub-planes of the astral realm can be similar to environments on Earth that reflect the lower impulses of human nature, while the higher sub-planes reflect environments corresponding to the highest notions of the soul.

In the astral realm, perception is heightened and unobstructed, with everything appearing bright and vibrant, as in experiences of lucid dreaming while in the physical body. Individuals have more clarity and are generally more aware of their surroundings, although, not everybody manifests the same level of awareness.

In this realm, sexuality has no significance, and matters of survival, such as work for aliments, clothing, or shelter, are nonexistent, as any kind of work is only meant for the evolution of the soul.

Individuals in the astral realm possess paranormal faculties as telepathy and foresight. Communication occurs through telepathy and the persons have the ability to see everything from a 360 degree perspective, as well as see through everything. Nevertheless, the enjoyment of these expanded faculties should not be a cause of entertainment and deviation from the most important purpose of astral life: purification, continuation of spiritual growth, and even possibly attainment of liberation from the chain of reincarnation. Individuals have the opportunity to more rapidly expand consciousness in this condition, which makes this period of intermission very propitious for spiritual evolution.

Since individuals transiting through the astral plane are spontaneously attracted to the conditions that reflect their qualities — by a phenomenon of vibratory resonance that follows the spiritual principle of like attracts like — they find themselves among other souls who are compatible and in the settings with which they are familiar and which offer the best opportunities for their self-expression. Each soul has an intimate soul group to which it belongs, composed of individuals at similar levels of development and with whom souls discuss their recent past lives, study, and help each other to gain greater awareness, under the supervision of their spirit guides.

When souls reincarnate their energies are divided, part of it remaining in the spirit world and the other part going to experience life in the physical plane. After physical death and upon reuniting with their soul groups, souls are slowly re infused with that part of their original energy that remained in the spirit world while they were reincarnated on a planet.

Because souls incorporate the seeds of the individual's inclinations and aspirations, on the astral plane usually they focus on the same interests as during their last physical life, and most of the time those things left undone in the physical plane can be accomplished in the astral plane, or they may appear again in a future reincarnation.

Thus the astral existence is up to a great extent delineated by the general make up of individual's desires and visions that may be amply expressed and lived out in a way that individuals can possibly abandon them by the time of rebirth to a new physical life on Earth.

In the astral plane individuals retain the predominant features of the last personality enacted on Earth and since the astral life is in many ways a reflection and continuation of the prior Earth life, some individuals will essentially have the nature of infants or children and others of youths or adults, depending on the age when their transitions took place. And all of them will differ in their attained world experiences but nevertheless be equal in soul essence and wisdom.

Further, departed individuals gain consciousness of their personalities during past lives, which remain in the background until the recent past life is evaluated and its experiences and learning integrated into the so-called "grand personality" that we are all becoming: the sum total of all the former personalities. This process provides us with a comprehensive sense of self, which is temporarily lost during each incarnation.

The astral life is a period of purification, restoration, and consolidation of all that has been experienced and learned during the recent past life in the context of other past lives and thus represents a continuation of expanding consciousness and evolution toward the Source. But individuals experience these possibilities to various degrees, depending on their level of evolution. While less evolved individuals are not fully conscious of this process, more aware individuals have great opportunities for further growth in the astral world that allows for elimination of components of the lower human nature and ascension to the higher sub-planes of this realm.

Free from the heaviness of the physical vesture, individuals can more easily unfold their noble, most elevated qualities. Also, intuition and inspiration are markedly enhanced. However, since free will never ceases, depending on the level of spiritual development individuals may succumb to longing for the physical life and thus remain within the lower sub-planes of the astral realm.

After death, individuals, provided they are prepared and are awake, reach a level in which they have the possibility of creating what was missing from their Earth life and thus indulge in their yearnings in the company of other souls already known to them. They may remain in this situation as long as they wish, but they eventually reach a time when they have satiated all appetites and have the sense that something else is waiting for them, prompting them to continue their journey in the astral realm.

Those who are not very developed spiritually undergo several periods of purification and evolvement throughout different lives until they accomplish liberation from the magnetism of the physical plane. This group of individuals experience such an attraction for the sensual pleasures of Earth life that, after death, they find themselves in the lowest sub-plane of the astral realm, desperately fighting to maintain their connection to the physical conditions of their recent life on Earth and may even reject the possibility of shedding the astral body, thus remaining in a very unhappy state.

Other individuals may find themselves in sub-planes where they are torn between attraction to conditions of their previous life on Earth and an attraction to spiritual life on higher sub-planes of the astral realm, remaining in conflict until one of the attractions prevails.

Still other individuals find themselves in astral sub-planes where they experience very little or no attraction to conditions of their previous life on Earth. They are able to take better advantage of opportunities astral life offers for growth and expression of the highest aspirations of their souls. Fearless and very active in their new lives they often achieve a full manifestation of their desires and experience joy and the presence of others of a similar harmonious nature. The more our life on Earth was oriented toward spiritual aspirations, the higher will be the sub-planes we may experience after death — or even while living in a physical body.

So in the astral realm individuals are confined within conditions determined by their own level of evolution, by their own limitations and in accordance with the Law of Vibration. While it is not possible for any soul to move into other sub-planes with a higher vibratory frequency than theirs, if they so elect it is possible for them to unrestrictedly travel to sub-planes of a lower frequency, with the exception of that sub-plane occupied by slumbering souls, to which only highly evolved souls are allowed free entry. Many individuals choose to visit lower sub-planes to comfort friends, or highly evolved individuals do so as a form of service to provide aid and guidance to those in the lower sub-planes. However, the majority of souls remain within their corresponding sub-plane, preoccupied with their own evolution until they are ready to continue their journey of ascent.

At each level of the astral world individuals encounter beings that are there to guide them, be it to resolve unfinished business from Earth or be it to become accustomed to a new level of existence or to help them make decisions about the future. In cases where people have experienced extreme pain and suffering due to prolonged disease or traumatic death by accident, such guides provide immediate help after death, by taking the individuals to healing places on the astral plane.

Healing and development take place on the astral realm by exhausting desires and working on mental aspects to cultivate abilities and refine the character features which are seeds that will germinate and manifest in future reincarnations. The entire process on the astral plane can be equated to what transpires through dreams while we are sleeping in physical life. In this case, the subconscious part of the mind, guided by the super conscious part of the mind, practices chores and receives advice, while the conscious part of the mind is not cognizant. The difference when souls arrive in the astral plane after death is that individuals may be more aware of the influence of the higher self or super conscious mind. Also souls in a discarnate state have possibilities of unfolding greater capacities than during life in the physical plane; for instance, compassion, love, and service can more easily manifest. In fact, on the higher sub-planes of the astral world only the more elevated conditions and emotions exist, such as pure love, harmony, serenity, and happiness.

Souls in the astral plane exhibit a central, or core color indicating the overall level of development and externally projected colors, or secondary colors representing dispositions and aspirations. After physical death, souls can engage in a diversity of activities; however the main one is the review and analysis of the recent past life as well as the implication of all other past lives. This is done in centers of learning (schools) and in the library, known as the "Hall of Records", both alone and with the primary group to which each soul belongs. The "Hall of Records" is where the "Books of Life" for each soul are kept. These books contain the sum total of events of all lives of the souls and can be used for study after physical death. This is what we know as "personal akashic records."

Other activities of souls after death are related to attending lectures by specialized teachers, learning manipulation of electromagnetic energy, helping other souls in need, aiding with the restoration of the energy of souls just returning after a physical life, and helping to balance disrupted energy on the planets. Also, souls participate in recreational activities and gatherings with other groups of souls, taking place in amphitheaters, gardens, or country side fields where they are involved in dancing, singing, and music and games playing. Some individuals need prolonged periods of solitude and rest; such souls are free to do not engage in the activities formerly described.

Sub-planes of the Astral Plane
These sub-planes are delineated by different rates of vibration and are inhabited by souls of like frequencies.

Lower Astral Sub-planes
The lower astral sub-planes represent the various conditions of consciousness that humans and religions depict as hell. Here souls are detained within circumstances close to those on the physical plane of existence, hence the term "earthbound" is commonly used to describe such states. Conditions can be described as dismal, cheerless, burdensome, foggy, dark, and cold. Here the astral body feels extremely heavy, as if made of stone, with slow movements.

A marked craving for the material life just abandoned keep these individuals in a lamentable state, where they reject help from spiritual guides and refuse to let go of their limiting beliefs, attitudes, and desires. These conditions are not intended as deliberate punishment from an outside source but unavoidable consequences of each individual's free will during life on Earth.

Consequently, such individuals are the creators of these wretched conditions, which can be seen as a self-created exile.

These sub-planes are usually populated by criminals; delinquents; people who have suffered from addictions; people who were sentenced to capital punishment; suicide victims; extremely cruel and hateful individuals; those who remain excessively attached to loved ones still living in physical bodies; average individuals who led physical lives too focused on materialism and earthly pleasures; those who experienced sudden physical death, be it due to illness, accident, or murder; narrow minded and prejudiced individuals; those who pass through the gates of physical death suffering extreme anxiety because they are leaving behind unfinished business; and individuals who do not believe in an afterlife.

Criminals and individuals who spent their lives committing acts of cruelty create astral bodies from the crudest materials of the astral plane. Thus, after physical death they remain in the lowest sub-planes of the astral realm until this shell disintegrates enough to permit them to ascend to higher regions. Their low and vile passions continue to exist on the astral plane, where they shape the appearance that reflects these qualities. So in these realms there are bestial and deformed bodies, since it is impossible to hide the true nature of the inner self, which manifests externally. Such individuals are extremely frustrated, and they continue repeating their brutal actions as long as their evil thoughts remain.

The individuals who during Earth life had addictions are, for the most part, unhappy and disappointed, for they have lost their physical bodies that were bringing them gratification, and they tire from trying in vain to obtain the same satisfaction. In their continuous wandering, they gather in proximity to the physical locations where their addictions were satisfied and try to influence living individuals to commit actions of violence and to continue substance abuse.

The individuals who committed suicide find themselves trapped within the same circumstances they tried to escape and obsessively repeat their exact self-destructive actions. They experience unceasing despair, suffering, and guilt. They clearly sense the pain of those left behind and then ask them in vain forgiveness. Sometimes they may not even be certain that they have died. They feel overwhelmed, as if carrying a heavy burden, and may also experience difficulty in forgiving themselves, since their act of suicide greatly delays their process of spiritual development. Moreover, it may be not possible for them to obtain permission for reincarnation for a very long time, and if they do get such permission the karmic consequences could result in them having some kind of disability, such as mental retardation, blindness, or paralysis.

Yet another group of departing souls may be detained in lower sub-planes of the astral realm due to intense affliction of ones left behind on Earth, which pulls the dead persons, while others are held close to the physical plane enclosed in a self-produced familiar setting, because of their own attachment to mundane matters or their terror of unknown environments.

Those who died suddenly and unexpectedly, usually find themselves in a state of disorientation and conflict, not realizing they have passed to the astral realm and are trying desperately to communicate with those still in physical bodies.

Generally there are two categories of earthbound individuals: One category consists of individuals who are yet un-evolved and thus belong to a lower sub-plane still very connected to the affairs of the physical plane. They refuse to refocus their attention toward the spiritual planes and, consciously or unconsciously, choose to stay close to the places of their former activities on Earth and thus exert influence over living people who have similar qualities, inducing them to perform infamous and cruel acts. Most of these individuals stay only for a brief period on the astral plane and soon reincarnate on Earth to be surrounded by circumstances which reflect their state of being. Nevertheless, no matter how short a time they remain in the astral realm, they always achieve some degree of progress. The second category of earthbound individuals in sub-planes of the astral realm are more evolved souls who either are in a state of confusion due to a sudden death or are unready to finally sever their links to the material world and therefore stay close to Earth, refusing to participate in their new astral life. These are often individuals who feel they left unfinished business on Earth or feel anxious about the well-being of a loved one on Earth. The individuals in this category are never fully awake, either in the astral realm or in the physical plane, and they are torn between two worlds, remaining in a dream like state of consciousness.

However, these earthbound conditions are only temporary and represent necessary learning circumstances for those who did not pay heed to natural spiritual laws and to the consequences of their actions on Earth. Because they did not learn their lessons during Earth life, they must repeat them until they evolve.

Although these individuals remain in an earthbound state as long as they cling to certain limiting patterns of thoughts and emotions and need to learn certain lessons, the time comes when they let go of these thoughts and emotions and ask for help in being liberated from their condition, spiritual beings are always ready to assist them in their transition to a higher state. When this happens, individuals fall into the state of soul slumber and they are later prepared for life in the new, appropriate sub-planes of the astral realm.

Because of their focus on their former lives, after physical death earthbound individuals may, under some circumstances, make themselves visible to those still alive in a physical body, trying to draw their attention by creating some kind of noise. Such earthbound people can also try to participate in the physical world affairs through the physical body of a medium or attaching themselves to living persons, a condition known as possession. They are able to do this when such living individuals are in a weakened state producing an opening in their electromagnetic fields, such as when people faint, suffer from debilitating illnesses, drink or use drugs, or become panicked.

Intermediate Astral Sub-planes

Intermediate astral sub-planes are inhabited by those discarnate individuals who were average and had very superficial interests on Earth; those who were somewhat more advanced in education and evolution; and those who were involved with world affairs that had a broad influence but nevertheless remained narrow-minded and selfish in their behavior, allowing their lower nature to rule them. Such individuals, after death, also maintain a vivid desire for physical life.

In these sub-planes, a larger number of individuals are fully conscious. These levels can be considered as astral reflections of the physical plane, with many similarities to it, although more vibrant, clear, and ethereal in nature. Thus there are luminous environments comprised of buildings such as houses, schools, and temples, as well as natural environments like gardens, mountains, rivers, and forests. Here individuals are surrounded by whatever they wish, in accord with their beliefs and desires. On these sub-planes of the astral realm, individuals have visions of their own "heaven" or "hell" created from their own consciousness. The more conscious individuals are, the more intense their experience of these "hells" and "heavens". More intelligent persons experience joy and grief as they clearly perceive the results of their thoughts and actions during their Earth lives. Thus neither "hell" nor "heaven" have a material reality, both being products of the mental patterns of individuals, although these conditions are very real to the souls.

Regardless of the experience on the astral sub-planes, individuals are always encouraged to progress spiritually. Therefore, their experiences should not be viewed neither as chastisement nor recompense but as essential aids for development of higher qualities. Individuals here, as souls, possess a clearer perception, can easily recognize the workings of the Law of Karma, and judge themselves according to their own conscience.

In these sub-planes of the astral plane, people reunite with relatives and friends who have died before them, spending as much time with them as they wish. They also have religious experiences. Those who are fanatical believers of a specific religion and are intolerant of other religious beliefs, form exclusionary groups in the astral realm and surround themselves with a religious environment that affirms the truthfulness of their own religion. Within these environments they experience whatever they expected, according to the teachings of their religion. This phenomenon has the semblance of reality to the believers, even though it is only a fabrication of the mind, — specific religious thoughts originating in the mind then create larger thought forms that perpetuate appearances on the astral plane.

Those who during Earth life were more broadminded and tolerant of other beliefs, likewise find confirmation of their views and see truth in all the essential teachings of different religions. Moreover, those who did not believe in an afterlife also band together surrounded by conditions that seem to substantiate that they are still alive in physical bodies. They also experience their own "hells" and "heavens" in accordance with their former actions, but these conditions are only temporary since deep inside each individual carries an intuitive knowledge that the soul survives after death, and sooner or later this knowledge surfaces.

Although in these regions the attraction for mundane things is already weak or nonexistent, individuals here still may experience influences originating in the suffering of people left behind on Earth, which may compel them to try to communicate with such persons, either directly or through mediums. However, discarnate individuals at these levels of the astral realm seldom initiate attempts to communicate with Earth themselves. For the most part they are very conscious of the evolutionary path ahead of them, and their main focus now is directed to various opportunities for a more elevated existence.

Higher Astral Sub-planes

The higher astral sub-planes are the transitory abode of the most advanced individuals, who led terrestrial lives characterized by service to humanity and spent considerable time in the pursuit of knowledge. Their astral bodies appear more refined since they have been already greatly purified by mental energy and spiritual work done during physical life.

These sub-planes mimic the intermediate ones except for being subtler and more refined. Landscapes are splendorous, and individuals continue pursuing the inclinations and goals they had during their physical lives, although they have a clear notion of possibilities of higher states of existence and eagerly look forward to ascending to them.

"Borderlands," "Hells," and "Heavens"

"Borderlands," "hells," and "heavens" refer to various states of consciousness experienced in the afterlife. While we live in the physical plane and after we depart from it we sustain our own states of consciousness ("havens" or "hells") in accord with the nature of our habitual emotions and thoughts.

"Borderlands"

"Borderlands", also known as "shadow lands", are states of consciousness after death where individuals find themselves due to refusal to accept the death of the lower ego personality and a strong longing for their recent life on Earth, prompted by a sense of unfinished business or by simply being conflicted. These feelings do not allow them to break free from their former life. Individuals in this condition experience dark, grayish, or foggy scenarios. Nevertheless, this state is not forever, and when desired individuals may get help from spirit beings to move on. Their condition can also be helped by the positive thoughts and prayers of those still living on Earth.

"Hells"

"Hells" are states of consciousness after physical death produced by extremely negative thought forms. Such conditions exist in close proximity to the Earth plane, and because their vibratory frequency is low they manifest as dullness, heaviness, and oppressiveness.

Individuals here are not chastised but only encounter their own negative valuations, principles, and preferences. They have to work out karmic debts and resolve misalignments and energy blocks. Here harmful habits such as fear, guilt, anger, arrogance, and cruelty, are discharged.

Individuals remain in this state as long as necessary to aid development. After changing their perspective and disposition, they abandon these realms, ready for further opportunities to progress.

"Heavens"

"Havens", or "summer lands", are states of consciousness after physical death produced by positive and benevolent thought forms. Vibrations here are subtler and faster. Light, beauty, and brilliance of colors are experienced in these realms to a degree impossible to imagine with our physical brain. The substance of these sub-planes is malleable and instantly replicates images conceived and sustained in thoughts. Thus, through collaboration in group work individuals create very beautiful environments which originate straight from their minds.

This is a progressive realm where individuals reminisce, reflect, integrate, study, assess spiritual advancement, and recall universal truths. Here people acknowledge and indulge in their capacities, powers, and virtues, such as charity, commiseration, love, forgiveness, tolerance, endurance, merriment, and bravery.

Individuals in such realms can clearly see the purpose of their existence as part of a whole in the context of their general evolution and take advantage of innumerable possibilities learning and developing.

At these levels of consciousness, individuals reunite with those they loved on Earth, including their pets. In addition, they continue to pursue the activities they loved during Earth life, such as scientific work, literature, art, or healing. In fact, many individuals living on Earth who are attuned to spiritual realms can receive inspiration from those realms and thus make extraordinary discoveries or create masterpieces of art. Individuals remain in such states of consciousness as long as necessary for further awakening.

Life on the astral plane is not only about experiencing states of heaven or hell as the consequence of the Law of Karma but also about experiencing the happiness of following creative impulses of the mind and expressing higher faculties and powers. Inherent within all souls is the aspiration to express themselves externally. This is a generative force that follows internal patterns and dreams of the soul, which may be more easily realized while in a discarnate condition. In these realms individuals can better focus their minds and more easily develop natural, specific abilities in preparation for manifesting such talents in their next Earth lives.

Astral life is very active. Here souls invigorate themselves while the process of growth continues uninterrupted, and everything learned appears in the next incarnation as flashes of intuition. Thus the astral life serves as a preparation for a more advanced existence in a future Earth life.

On the higher astral sub-planes that which is noble, dignified, and loving is amplified, leading to peace and joy. Individuals in the astral realm, especially those on the higher sub-planes, enjoy the company of those either connected to them by love, or affinity, or the same condition of being. These are much closer relationships than are possible in Earth life. Here a deep communion of like-souls occurs and they exist immersed in undisturbed harmony. Attraction and connection between souls happens because of similarity in vibrations and thoughts. Loneliness is not a possibility within these realms. Individuals in these conditions can also maintain links with loved ones on Earth, in the form of psychic and spiritual bonds. Such connections may be experienced by those still living on Earth as physical proximity of the dead person; while those who are disembodied, may experience it as a sense of somebody calling them or sending a message to them.

Summary of Astral Plane Experience after Death for Individuals with Different Degrees of Evolution

Experiences on the astral plane after death for individuals with different degrees of evolution can be summarized as follows:

Spiritually Elevated Individuals

Due to spiritually oriented work while alive on Earth, such individuals have already considerable purification of their bodies, including the emotional, or astral body, which has become subtler and more refined. They transit very quickly through the astral sub-planes since there is not much work they need to do here.

Evolved Individuals Who Led a Pure Life on Earth and Were Not Very Attached to Material Things

Such individuals require some time in the astral sub-planes; however, they remain serene and most likely unaware of their new environment until they awaken to life on the mental sub-planes after the various layers of the astral body are discarded.

Ordinary Individuals

Individuals in this group become conscious in their corresponding astral sub-plane, in accordance with the vibrations and density of the outermost layer of their astral bodies. They pass quickly through the lower astral sub-planes and their awareness is revived when they encounter stimuli from the new surroundings. Because these are individuals who have lived physical lives focused on amusement, sensuous gratification, and emotional exhilaration, their mental and emotional bodies are more difficult to disentangle. Among such persons, those who possess strong emotional bodies remain for longer time on the sub-planes of the astral realm, until the force of lower desire disappears by being worn out, and so the soul is further liberated. As long as the emotional body indulges in desires, its grip on the soul persists and slows the soul's journey. Nevertheless, in this manner spiritual growth can be attained, even if minimal. Since the emotions and desires of such individuals are still linked to their former lives on Earth, communication with individuals living on the physical plane is possible in both directions.

Un evolved Individuals

The allure of earthly material life has a strong hold on such individuals and their capability for expression is so limited that their time in the astral realm is short, and they soon return to physical life. Regardless, each one of their trips to the astral realm serves the purpose of eliminating parts of the basic nature and developing aspects of their higher nature. Their principal learning on the astral sub-planes is related to the development of a sense of fellowship and unity. The struggles they experience in a physical body are nonexistent in the astral realm, and given that the astral life provides unlimited opportunities to satiate any appetite they have no need for competition nor emotions of envy or resentment, fostering instead friendship, love and contentment. Such feelings are further amplified when such souls can reunite with former friends and loved ones from Earth who have experienced the transition of death before them.

Evil and Criminal Individuals

Individuals who led evil or criminal lives on Earth generally possess an undeveloped lower mind and they spend a long time on the astral sub planes suffering and longing for life on Earth, as well as trying to use any malicious means possible to influence inhabitants of the physical plane for their own amusement.

Individuals Who Experience Sudden Death

Individuals who experienced an abrupt termination of their physical lives due to disease, accident, murder, or suicide, either fall immediately into the soul slumber state or remain conscious. In any case, they are guided and instructed by spirit beings with the purpose of helping them to progressively understand and adapt to their new condition, making it easier for them to abandon old earthly patterns, but only if they are ready to ask for and accept this assistance.

Some of those individuals who remain conscious after a sudden death find themselves in their corresponding astral sub-plane, although they are not aware of the lost of their physical body and may stay entangled in the last scene of their terrestrial life; not comprehending that they have died.

Others may find themselves in an earthbound situation on the lower astral sub-planes, unaware of their death. In both cases, the individuals are unhappy, confused, and frustrated.

Individuals suffering a sudden death, who on Earth have led a life of evil doing remain earthbound, trying to connect at any cost with the physical plane, either with a feeling of repentance or with the purpose of maintaining their negative behavior trying to influence those in a weakened condition on the physical plane.

Ordinary people who die suddenly are, after transition, completely conscious and have the energy and desires they had during physical life but they also remain earthbound and confused, strongly clinging to the physical plane.

During sudden death, or the death of young individuals the soul is forced out of the physical body and the etheric body is thus hastily thorn away from the physical body to which it was strongly attached, causing it to remain with the soul and the rest of its vehicles for a longer time. Such individuals usually remain fully conscious and able to perceive the physical environment in the same manner they did while in their physical bodies because the former set-up of their minds did not have time to change and adapt, although sometimes they can enter a state of soul slumber.

People in this situation generally do not realize that they have died and continue acting as if physically alive, trying in vain to communicate with those still existing on the physical plane. The immediate consequences are feelings of being overwhelmed, frustrated, or in despair as they sense the suf-fering of their loved ones left behind.

In cases of suicide, individuals remain earthbound in a state of fitful sleep, caught in a vicious circle of never ending repetition of the same acts and prisoners of suffocating feelings of fear, hopelessness, and desperation.

Range of Post-death States on the Astral Plane

People have different experiences during the intermission on the astral plane, ranging from total unconsciousness to partial alertness, to complete awareness. These states depend on the individuals' extent of detachment from the recent Earth life experiences and their degree of awakening re-sulting from the magnitude of spiritual work done by them during their lives on Earth.

Nevertheless, consciously or unconsciously, disintegration of their emo-tional/astral bodies takes place.

The various possible states of consciousness of individuals on the astral plane can be further described in the following ways:

Unawake State

Some individuals, those usually less evolved, have very little self-aware-ness and are incapable of remaining conscious when out of the physical body, as they possess awareness only in connection with the physical form they inhabit. They experience an unconsciousness state in the astral sub-planes, without feeling or remembering anything, or even noticing their surroundings. They sink in forgetfulness and generally have only a vague sense of just existing.

Stationary Floating State

Some dead individuals possess very weak sense of self identity and have minimal alertness, apprehending their surroundings only vaguely. They usually stay at the physical place of their death feeling a floating-like sensation or feeling fixed to objects, places, or even persons and animals approaching the area.

Drifting State

Some individuals do not realize that they are dead and thus do not ac-knowledge their lifeless physical body or their new condition. They frequently wander around visiting places and persons connected to their previous physical life, believing that they are still living that life. They are somewhat alert and can evaluate their past life experiences to some extent.

Individuals in the previous three states do not consciously reflect on or integrate past life experiences, so they cannot participate in planning and preparing for their next reincarnation. Education and learning during the intermission are absent in these situations, consequently these people reincarnate automatically and unready, in many cases without any supervision at all. Frequently such individuals are reborn in places very close to the location of their last death and within a family connected to a former relative or friend.

Hazy State
Some individuals who have not completely released their etheric bodies as a consequence of either sudden unexpected death or extreme dependence on the physical plane, find themselves in confined spaces and surrounded by gloomy, nightmare-like situations. They are only half conscious of their physical deaths, of themselves, and of their new environments.

Obsessive State
To this category belong individuals who consciously choose to remain close to the physical plane due to their strong desire for worldly pleasures. They are aware of their physical death, but they try hard to communicate with people still living and even attempt to have earthly experiences by using those in a debilitated physical condition. Usually, such people cannot consciously plan for their next reincarnation other than possibly choose parents.

Mirage State
Individuals who during their Earth lives had fanatic and narrow minded beliefs about the afterlife are awake and self-aware after the transition; however, they exist in a dreamlike state created by the contents of their own minds where they are surrounded by exactly what they expected to find. Staying in this condition, they have no opportunities for further learning or expansion of consciousness. Commonly they reincarnate automatically without planning.

Awake State

Persons in an awakened state are alert, conscious of the process of transition, and pleased at being extricated from their dense physical bodies. They also feel happy meeting loved ones on the other side. In this condition of awareness, they can calmly evaluate their previous lives on Earth with the support and guidance of spiritually advanced beings. They can pursue their learning based on former Earth experiences, as well as new learning made possible during the intermission, all conducive to planning for the next life on Earth.

A mind which is agitated and perturbed with suffering, despair, guilt, fear or rancor, may very easily be an impediment for individuals to become totally self-aware and clearly conscious after physical death. The awakened state is reached through the evolution of the soul, incarnation after incarnation, until the time when the soul becomes totally self-aware and capable of recognizing others in the same condition as well as spiritual guides and teachers.

Transiting the Astral Plane

Summarizing, life in the astral realm is spent in one of the sub-planes, or passing through several sub-planes, depending on the new learning and evolution of the individuals, who carry the essence of all lived experiences. Along this process they experience gradual disintegration of the old astral, or emotional body, layer after layer.

Those individuals who, during planetary life, worked steadily and hard to lead a noble life and acted according to their most elevated nature have already done much of the needed purification of the emotional body by properly using their mental bodies. When such individuals arrive in the astral plane after physical death, little is left of their emotional bodies, making it easier to discard the residues.

Finally, after souls have spent the appropriate amount of time on the astral plane they reach a point they have sufficiently evolved so that their attraction for this plane has also being worn off. Souls are now liberated from their old emotional bodies and prepare to transit from the astral plane to the mental plane. When this happens, discarnate people shift definitely away from any possible attraction to, or influence from their Earth lives and become predominantly consciousness or thought energy. Since the mind is prevalent now, they undoubtedly know they are ready for the second death.

At this point the elimination of the astral/emotional body is completed and the individual moves to the mental sub-planes.

Life in the astral plane, whatever its nature and duration could be for each individual, is not the end of the journey.

Astral Shells
The obsolete emotional bodies released by souls are no more than residues of the seven concentric layers retaining some vestige of energy from the souls and are frequently called astral shells.

Such astral shells slowly gravitate toward the lower regions of the astral plane, where they eventually disintegrate totally into their primary elements. Meanwhile they float about reproducing, as automatons, familiar vibrations for as long as they possess remnants of energy.

Astral shells carry impressions pertaining to individuals' former lives on Earth, which are the result of constant exposure and response to stimuli so creating certain tendencies and habits that may be reproduced automatically by the astral shells and arise from old thoughts or feelings. Thus this apparent activity of the astral shells derives from the temporary survival of certain volitional impulses acquired during Earth existence. However, they are totally empty of life, will, and true intelligence. In addition, these astral shells exhibit a marked avidity for magnetic energy that they absorb like sponges and which gives them a deceptive aspect of liveliness.

Contacts may be established with these astral shells by mediums, relatives, or friends who mistake them for contacts with the souls of the departed persons.

Often, astral shells are attracted by familiar thoughts originating with loved ones or mediums used by relatives, absorbing their projected energy and automatically responding to it, creating thus a situation that is entirely illusory.

Second Death and Second Slumber of the Soul
Most desires of individuals are lived out in the astral plane in a very real manner so that the persons eventually lose interest in the astral plane and become more interested in the mental plane. Individuals sense that there is something else which still has to be experienced beyond the astral plane. The second death is the death, or shedding of the astral body and marks the point in which individuals move from the astral plane to different states of consciousness on the mental plane. At first, a gestation period is needed before becoming more aware in the mental sub-planes. So, free from the chains of

the astral body, the soul enters another rest period called the second slumber from which it later awakens with an intense feeling of satisfaction and joy. This second slumber of the soul is characterized by a calm, dream like state of being.

Life of the Soul in the Lower Sub-planes of the Mental Plane

The quality of this stage is also determined by the Law of Karma. Here the individuality functions as pure consciousness working as thought in the form of images and not as a mind working through a brain that results in words.

The mental plane is subtler and the vibratory frequency of its substance is considerably faster than that of the astral plane. This substance is also more refined and highly energized, allowing the expansion of the moral and spiritual qualities of individuals. Life in this plane is far more active, vibrant, and potent than the physical life and is imbued with a sense of peace and happiness, although the lower mental body is eventually discarded as well.

The first period on the mental plane is spent within the four lower sub-planes where forms still exist as thoughts concerning the personal self and is a period of letting go of old patterns of thought and attitudes. Here, thoughts are purified from emotional elements and erroneous beliefs are modified. Much work must be done with fears, complexes, memories of distress, feelings of isolation, and limiting beliefs. The more individuals can release these impediments, the more their consciousness expands and the more comfort and happiness they feel. There is no place here for selfish and wicked passions, hence they cannot be manifested within the subtle substance of these sub-planes.

This period is utilized to work on and integrate all the experiences and knowledge collected during the former Earth life. The individuals reflect on their experiences and evaluate them with clarity of mind until they understand their true significance.

Individuals are surrounded by light and harmony, and within these conditions they feel and see loved ones in their noblest ethereal manifestations, as images that become the living companions of the souls. Thus individuals can reproduce, with living mental substance, the images of those who remain in their hearts, and they so occupy their mental atmosphere, closer than ever. Individuals delight in the presence of loved ones for as long as they desire, as all desires are eventually satiated here.

There are no boundaries between souls, but instead complete communion. There is no suffering now, only bliss and oblivion of everything responsible for producing suffering and grief during former lives, resulting in tranquility, love, and pure spiritual thinking. The qualities of thinking and volition remain extremely active at all times, and individuals can easily manifest their creative nature through the power of mental impulses that are instantly reproduced in forms, which reflect the richness and strength of the individuals' minds, so that individuals create their own heavens with the best elements contained within their souls. Any limitations that exist here are self-created.

Life here is a sublime continuation of the previous Earth life. In general, individuals enjoy elated states of being that are the consequence of noble deeds performed during Earth life, and unaccomplished aspirations and goals can be manifested here. Souls work as creators of models for future material manifestations. Thus in this world, where individuals are less rigidly circumscribed and less deluded, they immerse themselves in thoughts, however they may still create their own illusions. Additional knowledge is also acquired here, and individuals are closer to Reality or Spirit, since they are now free of the illusory veils of the astral and material planes.

The length of time spent in the lower mental sub-planes depends on the mental richness of the previous life. If individuals have lived mostly instinctively, without developing many thoughts, they will not have much material to work with and will likely return to planetary life very soon after their emotional energy is exhausted on the astral plane. On the contrary, the more individuals have developed their minds during Earth life, the more thought material they have gathered and the more they remain conscious in these mental regions.

In the case of spiritually advanced individuals, stages on the lower mental sub-planes pass rapidly, with individuals staying in a dreamlike and peaceful condition to only gain new awareness on the higher mental sub-planes of bliss.

When all the mental material brought from Earth life has been exhausted, and the lower mental body gradually dissolves, its remnants are discarded by the soul. The shedding stage is now completed, leaving the soul absolutely free in its true realm the higher mental sub-planes, where individuals become aware of their Higher Selves.

Generally speaking, the shedding stage is accomplished in three different ways: First, individuals who possess predominantly emotional natures and have not sufficiently developed their mental aspects, remain a longer time on the astral plane until their astral bodies are sufficiently dissolved by being worn down.

Second, the case of individuals who knew how to maintain more equilibrium between their emotional and mental natures and who have endeavored more to develop their minds. They are more aware of the functioning of the astral and mental bodies and thus they can exert some control over them. In these cases the shedding of the emotional body is accelerated by an intense desire to shift to a mental existence. These individuals usually get in contact with the higher sub-planes of the astral plane and the lower sub-planes of the mental plane.

Third, individuals who are extremely advanced and have left behind the troubling nature of certain emotions and desires to focus primarily on the power of the mind, and are capable of bringing forth energy and light directly from their souls, easily eliminate the astral substance constituting their emotional bodies. Then, by purposely using certain vibrations –words of power— while guided by Masters, they accomplish the final destruction of the old lower mental bodies.

The duration of the process of shedding and whether it occurs in an unconscious or conscious way, depends on the individuals' level of spiritual advancement and the development of the emotional and lower mental bodies. In the case of more developed individuals, the shedding of the lower mental body occurs following an act of the individuals' will. These individuals are strongly connected to and markedly attracted by their souls.

4) Assimilation Stage

Now souls move to the formless regions of the mental realm, or the higher sub-planes, and remain absorbed within their causal bodies. The degree of awareness of individuals during this stage, again depends on the level of growth achieved up to this point. If individuals are transiting the early steps on the ladder of evolution, this stage is spent in unconsciousness and sleep, since such individuals do not possess powers to function independently within this realm. If individuals are more developed, they will remain more awake during this stage and this period will have more importance and a longer duration.

In this condition, souls are self-conscious and cognizant of all their past lives, as well as of all the consequent causes and effects set in motion by the individuals' actions during their physical lives. Within this state of freedom, souls can witness and better understand the workings of the Divine Creative Mind. They can also carefully evaluate, from a broader perspective, all the archetypes of form that evolve on the lower planes, and thus comprehend the relativity of phenomena on those planes.

Here individuals can form a strong determination to further pursue or avoid certain general directions in their next lifetimes. Further, individuals perceive themselves only in terms of their Higher-Selves and as part of a greater whole. The souls, free from the restrains of matter, enter a state of contemplation and focus only on their spiritual bodies. The concept of linear time —past, present, and future— dissolves, and the eternal now is recognized. This is a high state of consciousness, which eventually all individuals will also experience while incarnated in physical bodies on Earth, a condition achieved by withdrawing from the physical senses and freeing the self from the mesh of dense matter.

Immersed in this condition, it is possible to project the consciousness outward into multiple realms simultaneously and thus help others in need, or to have clear insights regarding universal truths and the unity of everything in existence.

The higher mind is occupied with abstract thoughts of impersonal nature and universal truths. After working with these thoughts, individuals carry them to the next physical life in the form of mental faculties and power, skills which they can use in actions during their new lives on Earth.

Moreover, the higher sub-planes of the mental realm are where additional development of heart and mind takes place. All the noble ideas devised during life on Earth, are further developed here and transformed into glorious realities to be brought back to Earth, by reincarnating souls, in the form of images with the purpose of manifesting them when conditions allow.

The mind, where thoughts are born, is the veritable origin of creation, and on the higher mental plane souls, like architects or designers, work to prepare plans to be used and materialized during future reincarnations on Earth —objective manifestation follows thought and meditation.

Thus, all previous attempts at intellectual advancement, development of morals, and service to humanity, as well as all other higher aspirations of the individuals during Earth life, are here assessed, transformed, and incorporated into moral and mental capabilities for future reincarnations.

This is an entirely mental and imaginary life. This is how the souls, during their inner period of existence, are learning to better live their next external terrestrial lives. All this activity contributes to the growth and development of the causal body — Manas — which will be transmitted to the other spiritual bodies —Atma and Buddhi.

While in these regions, souls may communicate with loved persons via attunement of thoughts, and vice versa. Moreover, souls here come into contact with more advanced ones and with Masters whose only purpose is to help the souls to further evolve.

The time spent in this state varies according to the quality of Earth life of different individual. In general, the length of time spent on the mental plane is approximately equivalent to the amount of content brought from Earth life that must be integrated as moral and mental aptitudes to contribute to the evolution of the individual. Consequently, the more noble, unselfish, and spiritual the lives of individuals, the longer they remain here.

Each subsequent period in the mental plane is richer and more expansive in terms of the knowledge received and the wisdom acquired. Thus, in each return to Earth life individuals bring a greater power and understanding of the natural laws of manifestation and evolution, as well as a clearer vision of their life's purpose.

The three lower worlds —mental, astral, and physical— constitute the pilgrimage field for the evolving human souls, the wheel of human life through which souls repeatedly return until their evolution at these levels is completed. The three "deaths" —physical, astral, and lower mental— are a familiar process to souls and are accomplished with increasing degrees of awareness as individuals develop toward perfection.

CHAPTER IV

Reincarnation, or Physical Rebirth

Reincarnation is a natural law related to nature and the design of evolution. For the soul to experience the denser material plane of existence, embodiment of a physical body is necessary. The purpose of being in a physical body is to learn and achieve total mastery of energy, and understand the underlying spiritual force. The main test for souls coming to planetary life on Earth is to overcome negative emotions connected to the fear and pain that is experienced while being in a physical body. This enormous task is impossible to attain in the short span of one planetary life, hence the need for reincarnation.

We know about reincarnation from the following sources:

— The direct teachings of incarnated mystics and spiritual masters.
— The teachings of masters from the spiritual world, channeled by apt individuals in the physical world.
— Insights originated in contacts with the soul, where the memory of former lives resides, often occurring during meditation.
— Spontaneous flashbacks to past lives, usually occurring more to children.
— Experiences in dreams.
— Hypnotic states.
— Using the techniques of age regression and past life regression.
— Research done on the subject by investigators as Dr Ian Stevenson,

Dr Jim Tucker, Dr Michael Newton, and Carol Bowman, to name a few of them. This research is conducted mainly with children who are able to remember their past lives, or adults under hypnosis.

Incarnation and Reincarnation

When incarnation into physical life is to take place for the first time, the individual soul extension, which is made of subtle mental substance and possesses consciousness, originates from the spiritual bodies or Higher Self or Upper Triad. It carries the three permanent atoms for the individual, which likewise arise from the Higher Triad as follows: The Atmic body gives rise to the physical/etheric permanent atom; the Buddhic body gives rise to the astral/emotional permanent atom, and finally the Manasic body gives rise to the mental permanent atom.

The Higher Triad of spiritual bodies is a reflection from the human Monad, or divine spark. Each Monad produces twelve Higher Triads, and each Higher Triad produces twelve individual soul projections. So the individual soul extension ready to incarnate for the first time would obtain physical, emotional, and mental bodies whose characteristics are appropriate for the needs of manifestation of that particular soul.

The soul enlivens the physical body by means of the etheric body for the entire duration of that physical life. Soul extensions have the potential to divide their energy into equivalent parts and thus experience parallel lives in different bodies and in different places if they wish so. Because of this capacity, part of the light energy of souls is always left in the spirit world when souls reincarnate in a physical body and is recovered when souls return after death. The main flows of energy penetrating the physical body proceed from the Monad (divine spark or real self) and they go through the spiritual bodies and through the individual soul extension, to finally permeate the lower bodies:

The first stream of energy enters the physical body at the top of the head and anchors itself at the heart chakra — this is the stream of life force. The second stream of energy penetrates the physical body at the level of the heart chakra and ascends to anchor itself in the brain —this is the stream of individual consciousness. Further, yet another flow of energy exists that connects the lower bodies, or individual personality, with the higher bodies of the real self, it enters the physical body at the solar plexus chakra and anchors in the brain —this is known as the stream of creativity, which is built up step by step through the spiritual work and growth of the individual until it constitutes that glorious bridge of light needed for Ascension to take place.

Diagram #1

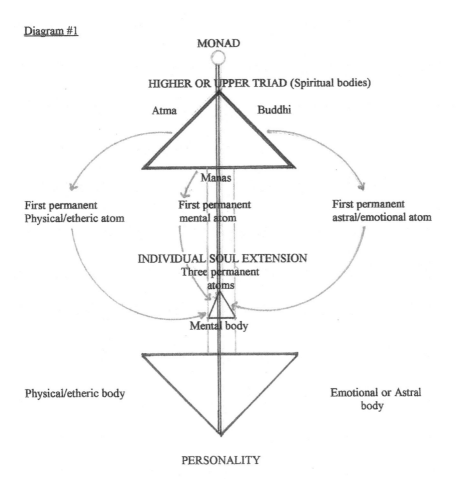

MONAD

HIGHER OR UPPER TRIAD (Spiritual bodies)

Atma   Buddhi

Manas

First permanent   First permanent   First permanent
Physical/etheric atom   mental atom   astral/emotional atom

INDIVIDUAL SOUL EXTENSION
Three permanent
atoms

Mental body

Physical/etheric body   Emotional or Astral
                                                   body

PERSONALITY

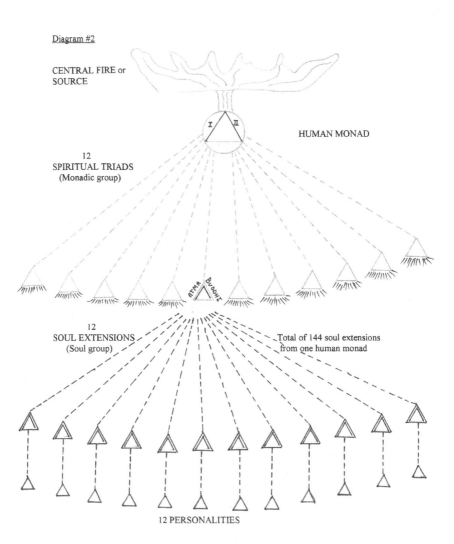

Diagram #2

CENTRAL FIRE or
SOURCE

HUMAN MONAD

12
SPIRITUAL TRIADS
(Monadic group)

12
SOUL EXTENSIONS
(Soul group)

Total of 144 soul extensions
from one human monad

12 PERSONALITIES

Personality and soul evolve together. During each new return to planetary life, or reincarnation the soul works with a transformed personality that is a coalescence of fundamental components of former personalities. Because essential aspects of character derive from the learning and experiences during past lives, experiencing different situations and learning new lessons during a life period results in new additions that reshape and improve the character of the individual. Character is perfected when individuals live lives in which, by using their free will, they choose to eliminate things which are harmful and obscure the nature of the true self, and reinforce aspects that mirror the divine image and consciousness.

Individuals reincarnate not only to balance karmic debts but to use their attributes and abilities in benefit of humanity. During the preparation time before reincarnation souls agree to take on certain task —a mission—during their planetary existence, which may be considered sacred. Later, while living physically, individuals may experience an exhilarating feeling of joy and purpose when they focus on actions that fulfill their secret agreement. Such people feel light, invigorated, contented, positive, and fearless about life and their work and activities benefit not only them but others as well.

By contrast, when individuals live without following the promptings of the soul and inner teachers, they have feelings of emptiness and lack of purpose. Such people hunger for power of some kind and look for it externally and in the wrong places, without realizing that their desires can never be satisfied in this manner no matter how prosperous their lives may become.

Once the soul reincarnates, communication between it and its lower vehicles is blocked, which is why the sacred purpose of the soul seems nonexistent. But in reality it is hidden to the personality and remains dormant until it is stimulated by the proper experiences of physical life and the individual is capable of establishing close contact with the soul. Important factors in assisting individuals with remembering their true nature and their purpose in the present life are interaction with others and experiences of suffering, pain, and frustration. Such experiences are like openings that may allow us to move beyond illusions and toward the awakening of our true nature. Our purpose in each physical life becomes apparent when we learn to consciously contact our soul and follow the course it has elected. If we do so, we attain empowerment and expansion of the personality and consequently of the soul.

Phases of Reincarnation

Human evolution, taking place in the three lower worlds —physical, astral, and mental sub-planes of the Physical Cosmic Plane— consist of the following alternating and recurrent phases:

1) A carnal phase, or outer phase of manifestation that encompasses the period from the moment of conception until the time of physical death

2) An extraterrestrial phase, or inner phase, extending from the moment of physical death until the time of a new conception.

The carnal phase consists of action in the world, while the inner phase consists mainly of reflection, purification, and reinvigoration.

The human soul is made of mental substance and possesses consciousness of self as well as perfect memory of every detail of experiences during its entire existence, including the successive cycles of its evolution. These cycles of evolution take place according to universal laws of nature, an important one being the Law of Karma, or Law of Compensation, or Law of Cause and Effect. Human souls have free will, but the process of evolution is subject to the Law of Karma during the carnal phase. During this phase of existence the actions of individuals are causes that produce effects that, according to the Law of Karma, result in debts and credits during each period of external life. These debts and credits need to be balanced under the impersonal energy of the law. During the inner phase, souls know that the laws of nature cannot be avoided and thus desire to return to the carnal phase to balance previous debts and credits.

The Law of Karma is not a punitive mechanism but an impersonal tool of teaching, which is set into motion by any action, be it mental, emotional, or physical. Progressing through the cycles of evolution, individuals learn, grow and mold their characters under the guidance of the Law of Karma. By expanding comprehension and realization, individuals advance and build up spiritual power. The proper moments for compensation, whether regarding suffering or joy, can appear during any lifetime to benefit individuals the most, from the lessons intended for them to learn. The places and means used are the most favorable for the individuals, to best help with their evolution. This law determines the conditions of our existence in both phases of the cycle of evolution. The links we create with other persons during our past lives, in part determine the family and birth place of our rebirth; and the debts we acquire toward others, contributing to either their happiness or suffering, are important factors in shaping the conditions of our next life. Often our friends of past lives become our family members in a new life. Resonance at a mental level between parents and their children is due to affinity of souls rather than to heredity.

We cause what is called negative karma when, through our thoughts, feelings, and actions we create a negative energy field of thought patterns surrounding us. Conversely, we generate what is called positive karma when we are capable of sustaining a positive setting of mind, thus creating a positive energy field around us. These magnetic energy fields then attract whatever corresponds to their type of energy.

Everything that a person projects in the form of thoughts, feelings, and actions while experiencing the physical world, is recorded in the ethers and remains as a permanent personal record for that particular being, known as the personal akashic records, or as "the book of life." Likewise, all deeds of humanity as a whole are also recorded in the ethers, constituting what is known as the collective akashic records. These records are available for review by the individuals to whom they pertain or by spiritual masters and the Lords of Karma.

The function of the Law of Karma and its keepers —the Lords of karma— can be equated to that of a colossal brain or computer, which makes infinite, invisible calculations destined to reorganize us, time and again, on the journey of our evolution. By understanding the mechanism of the Law of Karma, individuals can progress toward the aim of faultless attitude and action, as well as detachment from the results of action. So human beings reincarnate under the requirements of the Law of Karma and follow a natural sense of responsibility to complete part of their development.

Reincarnation is a universal mechanism of education and acceleration of the process of evolution, which every entity who exists on any planet belonging to any solar system in any galaxy has to go through until the time comes for ending these cycles of evolution by attaining Ascension. When all the necessary work during the intermission has been done, souls sense the time is right for returning to planetary life and, without a doubt, recognize the need for reincarnation in the physical world.

The souls have clear understanding of their karmic liabilities, so the general direction of their next life is then unfolded. In other words, when individuals are sufficiently advanced, they can elect their prevalent destinies for their new lives, including ordeals they will face and endure.

After a period of preparation and planning (when possible), souls are irresistibly drawn to their assigned places of rebirth and, following karmic forces, initiate the process of descent and re-focusing on planetary life.

The circumstances of a reincarnation, from historical, geographical, and family perspectives, are those which will provide the best opportunities for the individuals to accomplish whatever is needed for those particular life times.

Sometimes reincarnation happens almost immediately after physical death, while other times the intermission period can be longer and reincarnation thus be delayed. The timing usually depends on the degree of development of the individual. Because individuals are at varied levels on the evolutionary path, they are born under different circumstances, in accordance with the necessary lessons to be learned. At times, certain abilities acquired by individuals may remain latent during a particular lifetime to allow different faculties to evolve. Other times, reincarnation occurs under inferior circumstances because they are more appropriate for the necessary learning or for the fulfillment of a particular mission in a lifetime.

The Beginning of a New Phase of External Existence or Reincarnation
During the intermission period in the astral and mental sub-planes, the souls are purified and energized, far from the exhaustion of the physical plane life. At some point individuals feel the need to fulfill ambitions left unsatisfied during the past physical life, and souls thus are guided to reincarnate and reappear on Earth.

Impulses Leading to Reincarnation
The following five impulses lead souls to reincarnate:

1) Accumulated debts due to the Law of Karma.
2) The magnetism of planet Earth and the evolutionary process itself.
3) Attachment to material conditions and objects.
4) The inclination for self-expression within the physical world.
5) The wish to continue being exposed to the external world to increase self-awareness.

Thus, the Law of Karma as well as the desires of individuals are the leading force toward reincarnation. It is impossible for souls to reincarnate unless a desire for it remains still alive. As long as desire for something exists, souls will be attracted to those planetary environments that are most likely to satisfy them.

Reincarnation can occur either consciously or unconsciously. In the later case, individuals are instinctively compelled to reincarnate within the conditions that can provide the best opportunities for them to express, satisfy, and, if possible, eliminate all their desires. Whatever the nature of desire might be, noble or ignoble, it is always the force propelling toward rebirth and action in order to have, do, or be something. The desire to help others is as much a desire as it is that of satisfying our own needs. Every single desire does not necessarily have to be satisfied, for often the spiritual advancement of individuals makes them outgrow particular desires, which then spontaneously disappear. After experiencing many planetary lives, individuals become aware of the illusory nature of material desires and begin to feel the attraction of more elevated realms of existence, making it possible for them to terminate the cycles of reincarnation.

Elements Taken into Consideration When Planning a New Period of Physical Life

The more advanced the individuals, the more freedom they have in determining conditions of reincarnation

The following factors help establish the general conditions of a new reincarnation:

1) Capacity for learning.
2) Aspirations for a life.
3) The mission to which the person has agreed.
4) Existing and new relationships with others already born or to be born during a specific life period.

Second Appearance before the Karmic Council

Individuals to be reincarnated appear for a second time before the Karmic Council since the Lords of Karma must approve a new reincarnation, thus the accumulated karma can be evaluated and an appropriate embodiment can be chosen that provides individuals the necessary opportunities to balance a portion of that karma, correct past wrong actions and progress on the path of evolution. Under no circumstances must reincarnating individuals have to face more karmic debts than it is possible for them to balance in a given life period according to their level of development.

Thus potential life choices and different opportunities within these choices are discussed during these meetings, with the participation of spirit guides and teachers as well.

The frequency of reincarnation varies for different individuals, depending on their evolutionary needs, the situations on Earth, and the kind of people needed on the planet at any specific time.

Generally, individuals reincarnate in three ways:

First, less evolved individuals reincarnate unconsciously following the irresistible force of evolution. For these people, the intermission after death is brief, and usually there is neither conscious previous life review nor participation in the planning of the next life period. In these cases, new born babies may exhibit a distressful behavior such as being very demanding, excessive crying, lack of sleep, and anger feats, due to the fact that many problems of the recent past life may be still existent. Often this situation of fast reentry to the physical world occurs when individuals are focus mainly on the physical plane and unaware of the spiritual planes. Such children must be provided with a serene environment and special care to help them overcome their disturbances.

Second, individuals who are somewhat more spiritually advanced are more aware during the intermission period, thus achieving so further development during this time. Such individuals are more consciously committed to their own growth and therefore interact with spiritual teachers and guides of the inner planes, review their past life, and plan the one ahead with awareness of their karmic debts and a clearer perspective on their purpose and goals for personal advancement.

Third, individuals who are markedly developed experience a very active and conscious intermission period, during which they learn and work with the aim of helping others in need. They go through an extensive past life review and deliberately and consciously participate in planning their new life, which involves not only personal goals of growth but usually includes contribution to larger projects that aid the collective advancement of humanity. Such people assume more responsibilities and have more freedom of choice regarding new incarnations. However, these individuals also experience progressively less desire to return to physical existence and are more careful in selecting the environment of a future life.

Preparation for Reincarnation

After consideration of all that individuals have assimilated from previous lives, they make preparations for a new life, which involves selecting opportunities that will lead to learning and growth. To prepare for reincarnation, individuals are taken to a specific spiritual center corresponding to their particular Ray and are instructed by spiritual guides and masters.

During our past lives we have created karmic relations with other beings, thus part of the planning with guides and teachers concerns an extensive examination of the karmic aspects on which individuals should work during the coming life period and requires the participation of the involved individuals. Another part of this preparation process relates to having an overview of future possible physical lives with their main experiences, allowing so the incarnating soul to make a choice. Thus individuals are never alone along their evolutionary path.

Future Life Planning

The plan for a new and approaching life period usually begin with the choice of birth place, historical time, and parents, since this defines the setting in which individuals are reborn.

Individuals who are not very evolved do not participate consciously in the election of parents and are instead unconsciously attracted to parents due to vibratory affinity of minds. Conversely, those who are more evolved have the chance to consciously choose their future parents.

The parents facilitate experiences the souls need for further growth. Often those who will be the future parents may also be present during the planning meetings with guides and teachers, provided they are still in a spirit form.

The choice of parents is guided by taking into account the following:

- The opportunities those parents are able to provide in accordance with the general life plan and ongoing development of the reincarnating individual.
- The karmic links with one or both parents from previous lives, either of a positive or a negative nature.
- Appropriate genetics.

- The accessibility to a fetus, in the case of less evolved individuals who will be drawn to it unconsciously.

The conditions in which individuals find themselves at the outset of a new life period are largely determined by the circumstances of the moment of conception, the period of pregnancy, and the moment of birth.

The parents' frame of mind, feelings, and actions exert a tremendous influence on the newly reincarnated individuals, far beyond that of heredity; and that influence is felt even from the time of conception. If the attitude of the parents, especially at conception, is one of sacred reverence toward life and human relationships, and if they consciously desire to provide a physical body for the reincarnation of a spiritual being of high ideals, this will be the kind of soul attracted to them and the new body. By contrast, if one or both parents have negative or destructive thoughts toward the newly forming body, the soul pulled into this situation must balance its own karmic condition and help the parents learn something about themselves.

The choice of parents includes the geographical, historical, and racial characteristics of the environment in which the soul is to reincarnate. In addition, the individual is born when it is most appropriate astrologically regarding lessons to be learned, challenges to be overcome, and opportunities to express abilities and talents.

Throughout successive incarnations, the sex of the individual changes for purposes of learning and the choice of gender for a new life period depends on the experiences needed for the growth of individuals.

The next consideration is the part of karmic energy that will have to be dealt with during the new life. Then comes reflection on tasks and goals to be pursued by the individuals that will contribute to their spiritual development. These tasks and goals are both of a personal and a broader nature. The personal tasks and goals concern learning something specific and letting go of negative beliefs, attitudes, traumas, and reactions. The more individuals are able to accomplish the personal tasks and goals during a life period, the more they become prepared to use their gifts to contribute to the benefit of humanity, which fulfills the broader goals connected with their destiny. All agreements to participate in physical life, to work toward growth, and to help others in their development are made at the soul level before reincarnation. Often desires and determinations from previous lives influence the process of life planning, although they may be replaced by new ones during the intermission period.

Further, the individuals' inclination influences the role to be played, the type of work to be done, the goals for the new life, and the people with whom the individuals will be involved. So, inclinations, disposition, and aptitudes may continue from life to life.

The choices made while preparing the life plan constitute the combination of energies that will ultimately result in the physical body that will serve the reincarnating soul as its vehicle in the physical realm. Some individuals reincarnate with potential choices between various possibilities, while others return to physical life with a more definite mission. A life plan usually encompasses a portion of karmic debts, as well as a diversity of possible manifestations which would permit individuals to use their free will in making choices.

Later, after reincarnation, individuals are affected by this life plan in the following ways:

- From the subconscious they may feel impulses to either do or not do something, like getting post-hypnotic suggestions.
- During the course of their lives, occurrences significant in awakening them, may present themselves in the form of encounters with people, feelings of being compelled to go to certain geographical locations, or accidently finding certain reading materials.
- Through intuition and inspiration.

In these ways, the life plan of reincarnating individuals can cause them to make various choices that affect their life trajectory. Thus if individuals are sufficiently awake in the intermission period they can prepare the life plan for their next reincarnation from the broader perspective of their higher selves, following the guidance and advice of more advanced spiritual beings. In designing the plan, they take into consideration their existing qualities, inclinations, experience, karmic obligations, and areas in need of development; although this plan is only a generalized sketch.

Body Elementals and Guardian Angels

Blue prints of the etheric bodies of individuals due to reincarnate are prepared under the direction of the Lords of Karma, masters and guides, who also summon body elementals and guardian angels who are to serve the individuals.

Body elementals are highly intelligent entities who are members of the Elemental Kingdom of nature trained to perform the work of drawing and mixing material substance. Their task is to direct the building of the physical body, beginning with the process of first forming the etheric body following its blueprint, and then, during gestation to assist in the development of the physical body under the supervision of the Higher Selves of reincarnating souls. They will remain with the physical bodies until death.

One of the duties of the Lords of Karma is to assign the body elemental for each evolving individual, who belongs to the same ray of creation as the person. The body elemental stays with the same individual throughout cycles of reincarnation that encompass the entire planetary evolution of the person. During each intermission period after death, the body elemental and the soul of the individual are separated; one being purified and reinvigorated with strength, patience, and courage, and the other being purified and instructed about working on the evolutionary purpose. In serving the evolution of the Human Kingdom, body elementals expand their own consciousness and evolve in their own way.

Likewise, the Karmic Council assigns to each individual a guardian angel who belongs to the angelic line of evolution and remains with the individual for the totality of the person's evolution in the lower realms. The main purpose of guardian angels is to guide the attention of individuals toward constructive goals that will contribute to their growth. This task involves purifying the individual's consciousness with beams of loving energy whenever an opportunity arises, whether it is while the individual is awake or asleep. Guardian angels also radiate feelings of faith and optimism, using the power and qualities of the Rays of creation. The service of the guardian angels is part of their own evolution in developing right discrimination and wisdom.

These angelic beings undergo extensive preparation for their specific work of service to humanity and thus develop the attributes of endurance, compassion, tolerance, and serenity. They also possess a highly developed intuitive function and a strong power of invocation that they may use when help is needed from higher sources of power. They are created with the only purpose of assuming tasks of unconditional commitment. At a planetary level three lineages — the elemental, the human, and the angelic — evolve together, and although each one is on their own path they must work in cooperation.

The Descent of the Soul

When souls are ready to reincarnate they begin their descent into physical matter retracing their paths through the three planes (mental, astral, and physical etheric) and carrying within the three *permanent atoms,* which must be reactivated on each corresponding plane, thus acting as germinating seeds. The *permanent* atoms are infinitesimal particles that carry the complete information from all reincarnations. They are like recording devices that contain the total data concerning the progress of individuals in their evolutionary journeys, including the personal negative and positive karmic debts. Encoded within these *permanent atoms* are the choices and actions of past lives of individuals that will interact with the parental genes to define the dispositions of the new personalities of the reincarnating souls. As the *permanent atoms* are activated they attract the multitude of *life atoms* belonging to each particular individual, which were left on each plane and are now recalled to form the nucleus of the new bodies. Also substance from each plane is drawn to construct each of the lower vehicles anew. Thus souls on their way to reincarnation collect their own karmic seeds which have remained implanted in their *life atoms* and which originated in former lifetimes. These karmic seeds constitute the unavoidable burden of individuals.

Within our electromagnetic fields are retained the karmic seeds we sow during our different physical lifetimes, whether positive or negative. These seeds are gathered together within the *permanent atoms,* which bring back to us a replica of everything we projected outwards. In the structure of each lower body is one *permanent atom* correlated to it: one mental, one emotional, and one physical *permanent atom.* At the time of death, departing souls take with them these three *permanent atoms,* which remain in a dormant state until the rebuilding of the human bodies for reincarnation.

Thus, during the descent, souls draw toward themselves at each level (mental, astral, and physical) the *permanent life atoms,* subatomic particles of energy, belonging to them since the beginning of their existence in the lower worlds. Because these *permanent life atoms* are marked with the individuals' essence and karmic debts, they are repeatedly attracted to the same individuals by the Law of Karma and natural connection. It is the souls who are the determining source of magnetic attraction for the *permanent life atoms* destined to gather once more for the formation of new bodies for reincarnation. Also, there are *transitory life atoms,* those particles of energy which are periodically used and later ejected from bodies during our physical lifetimes. These are particles of energy that transit through the bodies of different individuals as well.

The new cycle of reincarnation continues with the revival of the lower mind as the soul descends through the lower regions of the mental plane and the *permanent mental atom,* or seed, awakens, attracting with its particular vibration the *permanent mental life atoms* and the mental substance, which resonates in compatibility and is necessary to build a new lower mental body. This first body to be formed constitutes the first layer of the soul's encasement and separates the soul from its higher world as well as affects the soul's workings. In other words, from now on souls will be working through the limitations of their new vehicles of manifestation.

Next the soul traverses the astral plane, and the *permanent astral,* or *emotional, atom* awakens the desire nature of the individual. Likewise, the *permanent astral life atoms* are gathered together and vibratory affinity brings about the necessary astral substance, forming a new astral, or emotional body. The soul is now enveloped by a mental and an emotional body, both possessing features and aptitudes already evolved through experiences of many past lives.

Then the descent of the soul continues through the etheric sub-planes of the physical plane, where the *permanent physical atom* is activated and the *permanent etheric life atoms,* in conjunction with the attracted etheric substance, create the new etheric body following the etheric blue print model previously provided by the Lords of Karma and Masters. This new etheric body is built by the body elemental within the maternal womb, and thus the seven central and main chakras, or energy centers, are delineated.

As we see, the formation of the etheric body takes place prior to the building of the dense physical body, which is shaped precisely like the etheric model during the individual's prenatal period. Once the new etheric body is formed, conception follows and the etheric pattern will be clothed with flesh under the joint influence of the body elemental, the builders of form, and the individual soul.

At the moment of conception, an energetic connection is established between the soul and the embryo, and a sort of etheric energy womb is formed around it. The consciousness of the soul connects with the newly forming physical body mainly through the astral body at first, and this link progressively increases from that point on. During the prenatal period, the mental body is gradually involved with the other lower vehicles, influencing the formation of the physical body and creating an increasingly close connection throughout early childhood. Hence, the soul experiences a gradual increase in magnetic attraction toward the physical body.

The father's sperm holds innumerable *life atoms* and, in addition, at the time of conception *many permanent physical life atoms* belonging to the reincarnating soul are psycho-magnetically attracted to the germinal cell of the father, which is united with the mother's germinal cell, giving rise to the child's physical body. Thus, the *permanent physical life atoms* of the individual to reincarnate are transmitted partially through the paternal sperm and partially drawn by direct affinity to the new physical body.

At this point, the psycho-magnetic aura of the reincarnating soul surrounds the merged germinal cells, and its energy flows through them. This is in reality, the monadic energy of the individual laboring through the reincarnating soul. Embryonic growth begins, then, by the aggregation *of permanent* and *transitory physical life atoms* belonging to the soul in past life periods and physical substance. So what we call heredity is not only that which is passed to children by the parents through their germinal cells but also that which always belonged to those individuals, namely the three *permanent atoms* and the *permanent life atoms,* which constitute a sort of personal heredity. Thus, in addition to the instructions contained within the genes of the chromosomes of the parental germinal cells, which guide the unfolding of the new physical body, there is something else, nonchemical and in the nature of spirit, which primordially directs the development of the physical body from the germinal cells.

Of paramount influence on the development of the physical body are: the etheric blue print, the reincarnating soul, and the body elemental, who defines the proper combinations of material substance and directs the growth process, remaining always near to the mother. The Law of Karma operates through the etheric body, the body elemental, and the imprints left on the *permanent physical atom* and the *permanent physical life atoms.*

Individuals, as souls, may exert an influence over the creation of their physical bodies growing from the parental genetic material. Hence, many times souls help to shape the new embryos, by imprinting unique personal traits through the radiation of their vibrations on the particles of matter forming the new bodies. This entire process is also followed by angelic beings and spirit guides.

The degree of development of the emotional nature and the mental powers in reincarnating individuals are taken into consideration in regard to heredity since the physical vehicle needs to be suitable to support the other vehicles, permit the expression of aptitudes, and allow for balancing of karmic debts. This is done through the influence exerted by the new emotional and mental bodies on the building of the physical body. Additional influences are the thoughts and feelings of the parents at conception and during the prenatal period and the behavior, mainly of the mother, at all three levels: physical, emotional, and mental. The more spiritually advanced a person is, the more the different new physical bodies will resemble each other.

Third Slumber of the Soul

The soul gradually loses alertness and eventually enters a state of semi-conscious rest and oblivion. Thus, in a way, the individual soul dies once more to the mental or to the astral life, as it did previously on the physical plane, and remains in this state of partial slumber even after it has reincarnated in a physical body. The soul then gradually awakens during infancy and youth, existing, in most cases, in a dreamlike condition during early childhood.

During the time of slumber, the soul assimilates all the experiences that occurred while in the intermission. There is always progress and change in the intermission period, and so the evolving entity is now a very different being from the one immediately after physical death. Many unwanted propensities may have been eliminated and many desirable ones cultivated.

It is also during this period of slumber that mental re-adaptation and spiritual preparation take place, all in anticipation of a new physical life ahead. Energy is radiated to the soul from its source, to invigorate it, and the soul strongly feels the power of attraction of its karmic bonds.

Pre birth and Birth

During the pre birth period, the reincarnating soul, linked to the fetus by an etheric energy cord, floats around the mother and usually moves in and out of the new physical body. The process is guided, stimulated, and guarded primarily by the Higher Self of the individual but also by other souls of friends, spiritual guides, and teachers, as well as the presence of the body elemental and the guardian angel.

The soul establishes itself permanently in the new physical body at any time after conception, the time varying for each individual. Although this usually occurs six to eight months prior to birth, it can take place briefly before birth, during it, or even after it. In a child's body, the soul has the ability to easily enter and exit the physical body until about the age of two or three.

During the gestation months, the soul's energy can affect the characteristics of the forming body, especially because of karmic influence. Similarities in appearance from one physical life to another, mainly facial features, are due to the power of the soul in influencing the growth of the new body each time.

In cases of individuals choosing to have a deficient physical body, for instance having congenital mental defects, the reason is usually to balance karmic debts.

Throughout the entire gestational period, the child is aware of and influenced by the emotions and thoughts of the mother, as well as those of other persons around, since three kinds of memory are now functioning in the individual: the continuous soul memory; the etheric memory, which is a sort of unconscious mind of the fetus at the core of the etheric body and which faithfully registers every impression of the embryo in regard to the mother and the surroundings; and the brain memory, which begins functioning at approximately the third month of pregnancy.

The mother's conduct is the main influence on the new child, affecting:

- The choices of the reincarnating soul.
- The maturation process of the embryo.
- The child's experiences during the gestation period, which will have a bearing on the personality of the child.
- The child's experience at the moment of birth.
- The child's experiences during the postnatal period.

Because embryos go through maternal experiences recording them as their own with the faculty of etheric memory, the manner in which the new child is received and treated by the mother and others is very important, ideally in a loving, protective, and welcoming way. If the mother has a history of abortions, has attempted to abort the present pregnancy, or just has thought of doing it, these situations may result in psychological problems for the child.

When the time for birth draw near, the etheric energy cord, linking the soul to the child's body shortens. Birth is usually experienced as struggling, many of the sensations being similar to those of dying, and the memory of it remains at a sub-conscious level that can be activated either spontaneously or purposely.

The process of birth occurs in progressive stages which begin with the experience of existing within an amniotic ocean and a feeling of absolute unity with the mother. This stage may be accompanied by images emerging from the collective unconscious, either heavenly or demonic ones, depending whether the pregnancy has been healthy or stressful. When uterine contractions begin, the feeling is of agonizing suffocation, or of being thrown into a tumultuous whirlpool, perhaps accompanied by demonic images.

Then it comes the transit through the birth canal, which results in experiences of asphyxiation and body compression, along with perhaps visions of fiery wars. Finally, at the moment of birth the baby experiences a feeling of expansion and alleviation that may have visions of resplendent light. However, the reincarnated soul experiences the restrictions of being encased within a defenseless child's body with the awareness of an adult.

Babies can perceive the entirety of their birth circumstances as well as sense the attitudes of the people present, and consequently these circumstances can affect children later. Further, during the time of gestation and at the moment of birth, many old traumas from past lives, especially those resulting from dying, may surface, stimulated by particular physical circumstances of the pregnancy and birth. For instance, reliving the sensations of a previous life's death by drowning or suffocation may be triggered by obstruction of respiration by excessive mucus; any kind of maternal hemorrhage can bring about a memory of having died from bleeding; and a long, difficult labor may evoke memories of a slow death due to being trapped.

Likewise, stressful deaths of the past that have not been psychologically resolved may result in birth marks, children may be born with skin spots or defects that correlate with the location of a mortal wound in a recent past life. Such marks are proof of the soul's influence on the forming embryo and may appear especially in cases when individuals are reincarnating soon after a previous traumatic death and have not fully assimilated the experience, retaining a self image from that past life. Such an occurrence happens mainly if there is a gestational or birth circumstance that acts as a catalyst to re stimulate the trauma. The memory function is strongly connected to emotions, especially if these originate in traumatic experiences, thus many times, after physical death, souls return wounded to the astral plane, retaining strong negative memories that may be carried over to a new life.

Newborns spend most of the time sleeping, and their souls, which still remain in a semiconscious state, easily slip in and out of their physical bodies, being more aware of the astral plane than the physical plane. This explains why children up to the age of seven, commonly when the awakening of the soul in the physical world is completed, appear to have psychic aptitudes. Once the soul is obliged to perform its work through its new bodies, it must struggle to completely connect with the physical body by attaining control over the subtler mental and emotional bodies.

After birth there is a gap in memory, the memory of past lives is nonexistent in the new physical brain, simply because the three lower bodies (lower mental, emotional, and physical) are newly formed for each reincarnation and did not go through those past experiences. Thus the recollection of past lives is dependent on the capability of our lower bodies to receive information from the soul. Such memories are stored within the soul memory, from where they can be retrieved only by connecting with the soul. This is possible when we are able to sufficiently purify our lower bodies, increasing their vibratory frequency, and we can divert our focus away from the physical world.

During the intermission period souls experiences and learning of previous physical lives are incorporated into an enlarged body of faculties to be passed on to another physical life time. It is not necessary that the actual memories of events of past lives be contained in the new physical brain, since that would only cause confusion and disrupt focus on tasks of the new life period. Despite this lack of direct access to such memories, many persons, through intuition as well as some vague sense of past lives, have some knowledge about the reality of life after death and divine guidance.

When the individual soul reincarnates its outward manifestation is the personality which is constituted by the three lower bodies: physical, emotional, and mental. The character of the soul must fuse and work together with the temperament of the personality; thus the soul takes on the challenge of trying to make this union as harmonious and coordinated as possible. Both, soul and personality influence each other; however, the supremacy of the soul must be eventually demonstrated.

At first, the soul contacts the developing brain of the child to learn its potentials in terms of the capability to think and sense things, as well as its blockages in neuron activity. During this important time of integrating and adjusting vibrations, the soul can exert its influence and stimulate the formation of the new brain with the purpose of improving its functions.

Continuity in Successive Physical Lives

Frequently, some characteristics of individuals and their personal relations may have some continuity in successive physical lives. If the mind is accustomed to generating the same kinds of thoughts in relation to situations, habitual thought patterns are created, which from then on become automatic and which can be carried over to the next physical life period. The same situation occurs when individuals carry, from one life to another, mental imprints that are the result of having suffered strong impressions due to traumatic experiences in a past life.

Continuity of the following may occur in successive lives:

- Similar physical characteristics of the face or body, as well as birthmarks may be found from one physical life to another.
- Certain qualities and choices, such as:
  Patience and understanding or lack of them
  Untrusting attitude toward other persons
  Abhorrence for something or persons
  Good or bad memory
  Good or bad temper
  Tendency toward rigid attitudes
  Spiritual orientation
  Extroverted or introverted character
  Certitude or skepticism
  Choice of nation, gender, and occupation
- Certain abilities such as:
  Leadership attitude
  Ability to learn a language from a past life
  Aptitude for the arts
  Remarkable intellect
  Ability for extrasensory perception or for meditation practice
  Highly developed intuitive powers
- Lifestyle inclinations (behavioral memory), such as:
  Addictions
  Yearnings
  Bodily habits
  Manner of doing everyday tasks
- Behavioral characteristics in relation to others, such as:

Inexplicable approval or disapproval of certain types of people

Reverence for, or rejection of particular belief systems

Effects of Past Lives on Health Aspects

Frequently sudden, unexpected death or traumatic experiences involving extreme pain, suffering, fear, or shock that could not be resolved can directly affect different levels (physical, emotional, or mental) of individuals being reincarnated, resulting in the following tendencies:

- Being overweight or anorexic as a consequence of having been overweight or starved in a past life.
- Having birthmarks as a result of fatal wounds in a past life.
- Having chronic headaches as a result of death by decapitation, hanging, or being shot in the head in a past life.
- Having psychosomatic symptoms or nightmares as a consequence of having experienced traumatic situations in a past life.
- Sexual problems as a result of having had a traumatic sexual experience in a past life.
- Not being able to adapt to a different gender in the present life—leading to transsexual or homosexual behavior.
- Having phobias, uncontrollable fears, urgencies, obsessions, antipathies, or complexes as a consequence of having developed them in a past life.

Objectives of Reincarnation

Reincarnation allows individuals to experience all possibilities in manifestation and master all lessons leading to the perfection of the human personality and God realization, which would be impossible to accomplish in one short period of physical life. We undergo innumerable reincarnations to experience different energies that bring us diverse lessons under the invisible influence of the zodiac constellations and the influence of one or another of the creative rays, until we assimilate every possible lesson and the entire potentiality of the soul has been expressed. The aim of all this is growth, from the lowest expressions of these energies to the highest manifestation of them. The process involves following karmic attractions as well as still unsatisfied physical needs and desires of the ego until the totality of physical life experience has been accomplished. Those in the early stages of evolution reincarnate more often due to a strong attraction for physical life. Some of the reincarnations may take place on other planets, when they can provide appropriate environments for an individual's next stage of evolution.

It is through these cycles of external manifestation that we discover that our destiny and only purpose is to unveil our true divine nature and comprehend that we are one with all creation and God, thereby reentering divine consciousness. A supreme longing for a higher state of consciousness must prevail to evolve consciously toward the revelation of a higher divinity within each one of us. This requires engaging in spiritual practice so our lower bodies can be guided by the higher ones to transform our ego-will into divine-will. Each re-embodiment is conducive to an improved way of living and new conditions for further learning. We always progress, even if only by an infinitesimal degree and even if unconsciously. Souls reincarnate in physical bodies, then renew their battle against ignorance and limitations and move forward revealing increasingly more of their divine nature.

As long as we allow ourselves to be driven by our desires, which may be interminable, we continue the cycles of reincarnation. As long as we remain influenced by the workings of the lower mind, the existence and the needs of the soul will be hidden from us. Thus individuals are engaged in an uninterrupted battle between their lower and higher natures while immersed in a material world, and remain shrouded in ignorance and continually try to deny the presence of spirit. However, this world of dense matter is illusory in the sense that it is not our authentic reality, and thus in each new reincarnation period our main task is to free ourselves from the grip of ignorance and illusions as well as learn to see clearly beyond the physical senses.

The cycles of birth, death and intermission continue, for us to grow, evolve and reach a deeper understanding of our spiritual nature and that of matter itself. Once we become more conscious of our purpose, we begin to approach physical life more seriously, taking advantage of the endless opportunities offered by it for our development, and this, in turn, accelerates the process of our transformation.

Growth occurs uninterruptedly all through the phases of human evolution: the external phases during reincarnation and the internal phases during intermission periods. We work steadily toward our ultimate freedom from the cycles of reincarnation by the victory of our innate higher nature over our lower one. This happens when we have an understanding of the transitory nature of physical matter and of the equally transient character of our evolutionary cycles through it; when physical matter exerts no more attraction over us but instead we are able to use it only as an instrument for the workings of spirit; and when we come to know ourselves as spirit, as pure energy that is part of a whole. At this level, we are no longer under the domain of the karmic law and we do not need to return to physical life unless we choose to do so to fulfill a specific task of service to humanity, be it in the form of teaching, helping non developed individuals, or bringing about something for the benefit of the world.

Result of Understanding the Process of Reincarnation and the Law of Karma

Understanding the Law of Karma and the process of reincarnation provides the following benefits:

- We take more responsibility for our thoughts, words, and actions since we are aware of their effects and their meaning for our evolution.
- We know we will have new opportunities to correct our errors resulting from lack of knowledge and understanding.
- We see more clearly the design of life.
- We can face apparently negative situations and life from a more positive perspective, knowing that every ordeal or challenge in reality was brought on by ourselves and is in the end, beneficial, since they only present opportunities to learn, advancing our level of development as human beings. In other words, we can more lucidly comprehend that during our physical life period we undergo various tests that are conducive only to our awakening, aggrandizement and betterment. The outcome of this understanding is that we are capable of encountering life with a sense of gladness, no matter what situation we are in. We also exhibit a supporting attitude toward the natural laws rather than opposing them.
- Assuming responsibility for our actions, we can better understand the apparent unfairness of life and realize that the inequalities and injustices have a karmic reason and they can be balanced along the way since our destiny is always shaped by ourselves.
- We gain perspective and become less rigid, less biased, and less intolerant as a result of myriad experiences during various lifetimes.

Each time around the physical world we can develop new talents, deeper understanding and clearer discernment. Increased opportunities for relationships make us less selfish and more capable of valuing others.

- We have less fear of death, and our increased understanding of the importance of remaining conscious during the process of death and intermission helps accelerate evolution.

Past Lives
The Apparent Oblivion of Past Lives

We do not generally remember our past lives. Some exceptions occur with children and with adults in connection with certain events or under unusual mental conditions that may re-awaken a recollection from the distant past. This forgetfulness is due to the fact that the three lower bodies —mental, astral, and physical— are newly formed for each reincarnation and they did not participate in those past lives. The present physical brain contains no impressions about that past. All that we inherit from past lives is an integral consciousness, which is the result of past learning and impressions, but not images and details. If this was not so, our state of mind will be too chaotic and we will not be able to focus on the new lessons and tests of the present life. This simplification allows us to use the newly assimilated aptitudes, originating from experiences in past lives, for problem-solving and for help in facing new learning situations in the present life. Thus, the fruits of past physical existence, which we bring to a new, are inclinations, characteristics, and abilities to be used in each following incarnation as part of the process of our continuous evolution, and are imprinted upon each new personality by the individual soul.

Each step in evolution, during many physical lives, eventually improves our ability to discriminate, make correct choices, and develop a moral consciousness toward all of life. For instance, individuals who spent many life periods committing destructive acts and suffering their consequences, at some point will gain the understanding that violence must be eradicated from their behavior.

Memories of past lives reside in the soul, and they can be retrieved by the individuals' conscious minds if sufficient sensitivity is developed in the lower bodies to make them responsive to the subtle vibration of the soul and with the help of a professional through sessions of either past life regression or hypnosis. This is especially useful when such memories might give us a better understanding of a present situation; reinforce something important that has already been learned; help us overcome blocks or solve problems in the present life that may have originated in a previous life. The objective of past life recollection should be to bring back to the conscious mind the essence of the lived experience. This happens when connection with the soul and higher bodies is established, since they are the seat of the memory encompassing the sum total of our journey.

Recollections of past lives occur either spontaneously or induced under certain conditions. They may happen spontaneously under special circumstances such as suffering from disease, extreme pain, worry, or anxiety; being in an accident; being under anesthetics; lacking food or sleep; or being in the usual awake state; in a meditative or trance state; using paranormal abilities like clairvoyance, clairaudience, or psychometrics; and during dream states. Another circumstance under which a recollection from a past life may arise spontaneously is that which is called re-stimulation. This occurs when a situation in our present life period strongly resembles another situation from a past life and this is then brought to the surface.

In addition, sometimes spontaneous recollection of a past life can occur because of the following:

- Recognition of a location, accompanied by specific feelings or visions.
- Stimulation by seeing an object, picture, or book.
- Stimulation by sound, such as listening to a certain melody.
- Recognition of a person whom we knew from a past life. This usually happens at the first encounter and either due to the eyes or voice of the person; or simply knowing it, having the sensation of some kind of repetition.

Past life recollection can be induced in the following ways:
- Hypnosis.
- Past life regression techniques.
- Programming dreams.

Some indications for the use of these techniques, called past life therapy or regression therapy, are:

- Persistent and disabling fears and phobias
- Constant worrying
- Severe depression
- Uncontrolled anger
- Blocks and inhibitions
- Serious problems in relationships
- Unending psychosomatic complains
- Serious sexual problems
- Severe eating disorders
- Addictions
- Severe withdrawal from life
- Mental confusion and feelings of alienation
- Sick behavior patterns

The techniques employed in past life therapy are the following:

- Inducing a trancelike state in the individual through magnetism or hypnosis, then giving suggestions and commands to go back to a pertinent past life.
- Inducing physical, emotional, and mental relaxation in the individual; guiding the person to focus only on either breathing, the pulse, or the heartbeat; then leading the person to imagine a given environment such as a garden, mountain, valley, beach, or sea; or to imagine flying, and encouraging the person to symbolically enter the realm of a past life by the act of crossing some kind of boundary, for instance a line, a door, a bridge, a river, a mist, or stairs, which may induce recollection of experiences lived during a former life.
- Encouraging recollection of a past life through the use of a physical, emotional, or mental link. For instance, a physical link may be a body sensation and the person undergoing regression is instructed to focus only on that sensation and even augment it, then go back to that situation in a past life that was the origin of the present bodily sensation. The same procedure can be followed using an emotional link, or a mental link, such as recurrent dreams, images, or axioms repeatedly experienced or used by the individual.

Past life or regression therapy can aid individuals by improving self-awareness about behavior, character, and life purpose, giving individuals opportunities to learn and progress in their current life periods.

Summary

As individual souls, we possess unlimited opportunities for evolution. All the latent endowments of the soul must be awakened through an experiential field and then demonstrated while in physical life.

Living in the midst of the illusions of duality, we gradually discover the laws of nature and develop our abilities for manifesting a pure mental life.

After each period of physical life, we return temporarily to the invisible worlds of evolution (astral and mental), during which time all the experiential material gathered during the former physical life is assimilated and transmuted into mental power. So apparent defeats are only steps toward ultimate victory; past errors lead us to increased discernment; past distress conduces to forbearance, courage, and patience; and finally all experiences are turned into wisdom. When the totality of experiences of one life is assimilated, souls are reincarnated for a new round of physical existence. They are directed toward the places, races, and families that provide the best circumstances for the development of the individuals. The new physical body is molded in accordance with the necessities of the soul, reflecting those limitations and capacities which need to be overcome and manifested respectively.

Individuals experience innumerable cycles through the three lower worlds (physical, astral, and lower mental), correcting mistakes and healing, each time on a higher level. The imprints of former lives, with all sensory perceptions, feelings, thoughts, and reactions, are contained within the non-physical, unlimited memory of the soul and higher spiritual bodies. These cycles go on until all possible experiences in human life have been lived and transformed into understanding and demonstration of our divine nature. In other words, until all possible stages of evolution, in each particular world, has been accomplished. Thus within this continuous flow of development and evolution, those who once where conflicted and struggling become the guides and intelligences of future humanities, and those who are more limited at present shall be considered as our younger brothers and sisters and their mistakes approached with loving tolerance instead of judgment and condemnation, since once we were also at that level.

Our thoughts mold our character since we become that what we think we are; at the same time, we are the builders of our own future condition and circumstances through the consequences of our past actions in relation to ourselves and others. This is how we progress and carry on our energy flow from life to life. Our interaction with others creates certain bonds, either of love or of rejection. Those bonds of love are reinforced during each new life, be it on the physical realm or during intermission in the inner worlds; and those of rejection end and liberate us when we become wise enough to let them go.

We just wear masks and costumes each time to play a different illusory role and dance the dance of creation on the physical realm that always serves our purpose of evolution. During this process we are never alone; we are always aided and guided by those from humanity who have already evolved further and by high spiritual intelligences.

Nevertheless, I should mention that this sequential occurrence of our innumerable lifetimes it is so only from the perspective of sluggish linear time, or how we perceive and understand it with a three-dimensional consciousness. Thus the chronological order of our different incarnations is part of the grand illusion at these levels of manifestation, while from the higher perspective of spirit, all these lifetimes are in reality happening in unison within the perpetual now.

Beyond Reincarnation

Moreover, planet Earth is only one of the countless experiential fields of the cosmos where some of the stages of human evolution take place.

Once individuals have reached a certain point in this spiritual evolution, they have liberated from the chain of reincarnations and experience ascension. Now individuals have a clear knowledge of their true nature and their connection to the greater whole. Now individuals have awakened, their hearts are expanded, and they access true wisdom. But this does not signify an end point in evolution since there is an infinite range of levels of existence, world after world, through which the human spiritual entities shall still transit.

Some Distinctions

Three conditions must be separated from the concept of reincarnation since they are not part of it. The first is the condition known as "walk in". This condition refers to a human soul, other than the original owner of a particular physical body, appropriating that body, which is usually the body of a child, or more exceptionally the body of an adult. It is a mutual agreement to exchange souls: one goes out, another comes in. Generally, this can happen while a person is suffering from a severe illness and most of the times results in a notorious change in the personality of the individual after recovery. The second condition is known as "identification". This may happen when dying individuals are incapable of completely letting go of material existence and during the intermission period they remain in a dreamlike condition, imagining they are still part of the physical landscape as a plant, a rock, an animal, an object, or even another living person to whom they attach and totally identify.

The third condition is known as "overshadowing". This is also an agreement between two souls, by which one of them "overshadows" the other taking complete command of the lower bodies of that soul, with the higher purpose of accomplishing special missions. The overshadowing soul is always the soul of a spiritual master.

CHAPTER V

Preparation for a Good Death

Changing Our Attitude toward Life and Death

How we experience the process of death reflects our habitual tendencies during physical life, whether they are positive or negative in nature.

To be well prepared for the transition of death we must modify our attitude to living and thus death, in the various ways discussed in the following sections.

Learning to Look at the World and Ourselves as Being in Perpetual Change and Transformation

To be properly prepared for the transition of death, we must accept change in life. Change is the very essence of nature, in front of our eyes all the time, even if we try to ignore it. We must see our reality as it truly is and work with change instead of antagonizing it or trying to evade it. When we modify our behavior and release harmful patterns we are changing ourselves for the better, which enhances freedom, happiness, and confidence. We must learn from change, flow with it, and let go of attachments. This welcoming attitude toward change allows us to accost the transition of death with acceptance and even a sense of adventure.

Living Life with the Energy of Love, Joy, and Gratitude

Love is a primordial determinant in the process of death. Depending on how much love we feel and demonstrate during physical life, will be our condition at the moment of death and thereafter.

Being able to maintain positive thinking at the moment of death is extremely important to our circumstances following this transition. If we create the habit of positive thinking during our lives, in the face of any circumstance, we will spontaneously have positive thoughts at the moment of death. A solid positive imprint on the mind at this time is of vital importance, because it leads to equally positive circumstances during the intermission period and the following reincarnation.

Also it is crucially important to live with a joyful attitude and infuse our lives with meaning and gratitude to be properly prepared for death and face it with no regrets. If we believe we are not capable of maintaining a positive attitude during death we can seek assistance from another person who can guide us.

Living a Life Free of Fears
Learning to eliminate fears in our lives prepares us to conquer the great fear of death as well.

Connecting with our inner wisdom for guidance and knowledge helps us to overcome fears. One means of establishing such a connection is meditation, which leads to the experience of oneness with all life, which is God. Further, bravely confronting our own mortality while living prepares us to face death fearlessly and also helps us to deal with fears while living, allowing us to experience physical life in a far more profound, joyful, and productive manner.

Living a Life Free of Stress
When we learn about the supremacy of our mental over our physical and emotional natures and we gain control of our mind, we can orient our mind to positive thoughts and create the habit of having a calm mind, which entails relaxation. If this condition is familiar to us, when the moment of death approaches we will be able to face it calmly.

Living with the Purpose of Spiritual Development and Sustaining Connection with the Divine
Living with the purpose of spiritual growth can prepare us to face death fearlessly since we learn to see it only as a continuation of a process and not as the end of our being. To live in this manner we need to explore our inner selves. We can best do this during frequent periods of being alone and through meditation and contemplation to discover our true selves, the nature

of life and death, and the purpose of our life. Only by observing ourselves profoundly can we understand our mission for a given life period.

The practice of meditation can discipline us to control our minds, which is especially useful during the process of death, when it is advantageous to be able to recognize the various mental projections that take place then and to let them guide us to higher spiritual realities.

When we consciously seek spiritual advancement we learn to live with greater awareness, lose our fear of death and reach a point where we master the transition of death. Through spiritual work we come out of ignorance and move toward the luminosity of the soul, and then physical death is divested of the threatening meaning we usually assign to it.

If we are capable of maintaining a heartfelt link to the energy we call God at all times, learning to shift our perception from identification with a physical body to seeing ourselves as living souls, we know we are part of that energy, therefore compassion and love are with us and there is no place for fear of any kind, including the fear of death.

Developing and Sustaining Faith

Faith arises from the knowledge that we are part of that encompassing energy which is Life or God and that our true essence cannot ever be exterminated. Sustaining this faith before and at the moment of death brings peace, reassurance, and a sense of connection with humanity and universal energy.

Cultivating Acceptance of Death

Creating the habit of repeatedly meditating and pondering about death in general, as well as our own death in particular, eventually gives us a deep understanding of the intrinsic association between life and death. As a result, we learn to accept death as something natural, not threatening, and a part of the larger process of perpetual living.

By truly accepting death, which is unavoidable anyway, we become less attached to physical life and can more clearly see the benefits of preparing ourselves for the moment of death while we are still living.

Cultivating Happiness toward Death

We can accomplish this by first realizing how dying is in reality the return of substance that we have utilized to manifest, and thus experience physical life, to its original source. In other words, we give back that which we temporarily needed: a physical, an emotional, and a mental body. Second, by feeling gratitude in our heart for the innumerable possibilities we have been given to progress spiritually in each physical life period; and finally, understanding death as a momentary liberation of our soul from the burdens and restrictions of physical existence.

If we can reach such profound level of understanding, both death and life take on a different meaning — that of a continuum, experienced as we evolve. Thus we reach a point where there is no suffering, no apprehension, and no dread at the thought of death. So, changing our attitude toward life make us also change our attitude toward death, and this induces us to want to approach it properly, for which we must prepare and develop goals.

The Ideal Approach to Death
Death, which is a supremely important and powerful moment in the process of living since it offers not only possibilities for spiritual growth but even for liberation from the cycles of reincarnation, ideally should be faced in the following manner:

- With complete consciousness, without sedation of any kind. In this manner dying becomes a conscious act and our soul can withdraw from the physical body quickly.
- With knowledge of the process of dying, so we can better use those opportunities offered for either attaining higher states of consciousness or for total liberation.
- Knowing that death is the pinnacle of a physical life period and only part of a continuum of life.
- With a welcoming, relaxed attitude.
- With pure and positive thoughts.
- Calmly, without fear and with a spirit of adventure and gladness, to avoid recoiling to lower states of consciousness.
- With dignity rather than as a victim.
- Focusing on a beautiful image of nature, such as the sky, or the sun; or focusing on a spiritual teacher or enlightened being to direct the self identity beyond that of the human ego and toward higher aspects of reality.
- In a state of devotion which can be done by repeating a prayer, a

mantra, an affirmation, the name of God or an enlightened person, as a means of purification and focus on higher levels of consciousness.

- In the company of aware and supportive people.
- With the help of a guiding person or "support person" who gives commands, either verbally or mentally, to remind the dying persons of the steps in the process of death, helping them to merge with the Light and accept it as their own divine nature and supreme reality.

The ideal way of facing death for those who surround or are close to the dying is the following:

- Knowing about the death process and accepting it without resistance.
- Having sacred respect for death.
- Having a positive perspective and praying.
- Maintaining an attitude of serenity, kindness and love.
- With a selfless spirit of helping the dying individuals in their departure from the physical world.

Goals for the Process of Death

If we can attain the following goals at the time of death we will transform the experience of death from a fearful agonizing departure to an ecstatic and liberating transition:

- To die knowledgeable of what the process of death involves.
- To die in a state of peace and devotion.
- To die with full consciousness, totally present and aware, and know it is not a dream.
- To completely let go our dualistic material, emotional, and mental habits with absolute trust in the new developments ahead.
- To avoid being detained in the gray zone lost in a state of confusion, which may occur if experiencing terror or shock.
- Not to avoid the various visions and sounds of the death process, knowing they are reflections of our mind and are ultimately benevolent in nature.
- To have a good rebirth in the immediate intermission period and in the next life period by following the brighter lights and not the dimmer ones at the moment of death.

- To attain liberation from the cycles of physical reincarnation by being able to totally merge with the resplendent and powerful Light of absolute consciousness, recognizing it as our own essence.

Preparation for Physical Death

The manner in which we are currently living influences the circumstances of our future. The present life period is the time to transform our future by making positive changes in our current lives and preparing for our encounter with death.

<u>Practical Preparation</u>

We can prepare for death practically by facing our mortality and taking the following steps to ensure practical matters will not undermine serenity at the time of death:

- Making sure all our material matters are in order. In doing this we prepare ourselves for the best and fastest departure by eliminating reasons that may keep us tethered to the material plane resisting letting go.
- Ending discord with others, either personally or mentally, by releasing our resentments to attain serenity.
- Saying goodbye to everything and everybody.
- Contemplating arranging for cremation, since this procedure accelerates the return of the physical atoms to their original source and also it helps to diminish the natural attraction of the human soul for its physical body.
- Rejecting autopsy or embalming in order to aid the soul with a peaceful withdrawal from the physical body.

<u>Mental Preparation</u>

The intellectual part of the mind is the agent for knowledge and eventually one of the means for liberation. We can prepare for death mentally by acquiring knowledge throughout our life period about the process of death by reading and studying spiritual teachings, then creating in our minds vivid scenes of what can be expected at the time of death and working to understand it. We can practice remembering these images periodically and thus cultivate the habit of thinking about and accepting our own mortality.

Ideally we should promote familiarity with physical death from an early age, thus we will be ready to go through the transition of death calmly when the time comes.

It is also important to develop our faculty of imagination by practicing creative imagining of ideal scenarios for the death moment and possible realms of existence with beautiful landscapes immediately following death. Such practice makes us familiar with the different situations we may face after death and thus reinforces our self-confidence.

Emotional and Moral Preparation

We can prepare for death emotionally and morally by modifying living habits as follows:

- Living in a more profound and intense manner.
- Living in a more enjoyable way and creating joy for others by practicing acceptance, tolerance, sensitivity, compassion, and generosity.
- Being more at ease in relationships, remembering their transient nature and giving them the most positive energy possible.
- Being more at ease with our physical body, caring for it without becoming unnecessarily preoccupied about it.
- Observing ourselves and discovering our propensity toward negative emotions and thoughts in order to transform our reactions and condition our mind for positive thinking. For instance, working in transmuting impatience into patience and anger into tolerance.
- Disengaging from things we tend to cling too excessively.
- Detaching ourselves from things which belong to us by giving them away.
- Cultivating acceptance and welcoming changes in our lives, as well as an attitude of open-mindedness to problems.

Using Sleep and Dreams to Better Understand Death

Observing the stages we go through during sleep and the nature of our dreams can help us prepare for death. By doing this we can realize that there are correlations between this process and the process of dying. The moment of death and the melting of the elements correspond with falling asleep, and dreaming corresponds with the experiences of the intermission period after death. To learn more about such parallels we can think about the moment of death and enact it each time we fall asleep, trying to follow the different stages of the death process.

Working with our dreams play a crucial role in our preparation for physical death since it can help us tremendously in keeping an unbroken, clear state of consciousness during and after death. We can use the sleep time as a practice for death to become consciously acquainted with the possible scenarios occurring during and after physical death. Further, by practicing lucid dreaming, which entails complete self-awareness within a dream with clear knowing that we are dreaming, we will be rehearsing our circumstances during the intermission period. This practice prepares us for acknowledging our situation, without confusion, when we actually are in the intermission period after death.

The manner in which we behave in different life situations and in the face of obstacles, as well as our reactions in dreams and nightmares gives us a hint of how we will react to various scenarios after death. Being aware of this we can favorably adjust our behavior before death.

The goal of these practices is accomplishing mastery over the various realms of the mind, which reflect different states of consciousness.

Engaging in Spiritual Practices

We can also prepare ourselves for the transition of death through spiritual practices that help us learn to balance and control thoughts and emotions, which could otherwise cause overwhelming situations, and assist us in gaining knowledge of connection to spirit.

The following types of spiritual practices can be helpful for these purposes:

- Meditation: This practice, which helps us work with our breath by following it with awareness, teaches us about relaxation and letting go of stress, which prepares us for the ultimate letting go of Earth life at the moment of death; teaches us about the predominance of mind and about developing one pointed focus, transferring it to higher spiritual realities; brings us peace and clarity about ourselves; detachment from thoughts and emotions; consciousness; expands the self and exposes us to inner lights and sounds that make us more familiar with such experiences during the process of death.
- Conscious Association of Daily Tasks with Spiritual Practice: This practice is done by aligning ordinary daily activities with spirituality.

Thus washing becomes cleansing of negativity; walking becomes a prayer of gratitude; opening a door or a window becomes a welcoming of wisdom; talking becomes sacred communication, and so on.

- Expanding the Heart Chakra: This practice involves visualizing green and pink lights coming from above and entering the body through the Crown Chakra then directing the lights down to the Heart Chakra and letting them spin in a circle, expanding it more and more until it encompasses the entire universe, and remaining within this feeling as long as possible.
- Prayers: This practice focuses on invoking spiritual beings and teachers for strength and illumination, or as a means of expressing devotion and gratitude.
- Repetition of Mantras or Positive Affirmations: This practice involves maintaining a focused mind, invoking higher states of consciousness by repeating a mantra such as "OM MANI PADME HUM" (mantra of great compassion and purification of body, speech, and mind) or simply "OM", or positive affirmations like "I am one with God"; "I am one with... (Name of a master); "I am love"; "I am spirit"; or "I am soul".
- Reflecting on Love: This practice involves reflecting on love as our link with other beings and all existence, therefore it opens and expands the Heart Chakra.

Exercises to Prepare for Death

Breathing Exercise

This exercise allows us to associate death with relaxation and letting go, helping to diminish the fear of death. The main focus of attention during this exercise should be on the exhalation.

- With closed eyes take a deep breath.
- With total consciousness, breathe out slowly, letting go of everything as at the moment of death.
- Maintain an embracing attitude while continuing to breathe in this manner.

Breathing While Repeating Affirmations

- With closed eyes focus completely on the breath.

- Inhale deeply while thinking: "I know I am aging."
- Exhale slowly while thinking: "I know I cannot avoid it."
- Inhale deeply thinking: "I know I will die."
- Exhale slowly thinking: "I know I cannot avoid it."
- Inhale deeply thinking: "I know there would be a time when I have to leave all that I love."
- Exhale slowly thinking: "I know I cannot avoid it."
- Inhale deeply thinking: "I know my consciousness is deathless."
- Exhale slowly thinking: "I am calm and joyful."

Breathing and Expanding the Body
- With closed eyes, inhale deeply and feel that your body expands.
- Exhale slowly and let go of everything.
- With each new inhalation your body expands further and gets larger and larger.
- Remain with this feeling as long as you can.

Visualization Exercises
Visualizing in the mind or actually looking at strong sources of light can help us to be prepared for the encounter with the inner lights at death. The following are some ways to practice this:

- Visualize the sun in your mind, view a picture of it, or actually look at it indirectly or with dark glasses.
- Look at a light bulb and keep concentrating on it. Different colors of light bulbs can be used.
- Look intently at a picture of a mandala or an enlightened person of your choice and retain a memory of the individual's features. Then, with closed eyes try to recall the image in your mind, holding it as long as possible.

Creative Imagination Exercises
- Imagine that you are at the moment of your death. Examine your attitudes and actions during your life to discover any remorse, determine what modifications you can make to avoid it, and to complete any unfinished tasks.
- Imagine that you are visiting the other side and use a portal to gain

access to it, such as a door, path, bridge, or stairs. Then imagine a location where you encounter a teacher for guidance. Return to your present life with the resolve to live differently, for instance, with more courage, determination, love, and compassion.

- Lying down, with closed eyes, imagine your own death, funeral, and burial or cremation.
- Lying down with closed eyes, imagine that you are dead and simply observe yourself, without identifying with anything. First focus on your feet, imagining that they are in flames. Then imagine the fire progressing upwards, consuming each part of your body — your legs, trunk, arms, hands, neck, and finally your head — until your whole body is burning; becoming ashes, and slowly disappearing. Remain calm as only a witness, realizing that you are not your physical, your emotional, or your lower mental bodies.
- Lying down with closed eyes and remaining detached as only an observer, imagine that you are dead. See and feel your body melting away until only your skeleton remains.

Practicing the Moment of Death

The purpose of this exercise is to learn how to be fully prepared when the moment of death arrives, including being conscious of what is happening; not succumbing to shock and fear; being able to be alert during the entire process and so find an easier and faster way through it, accelerating the final departure from the physical body. This practice forces us to face the suffering and fear caused by the idea of ceasing to exist, leading us to discover that we do not stop existing and so we should not fear death.

When we regularly practice this process, we will be well trained in appropriate reflexes and responses if sudden, unexpected death should occur. Additional positive results derived from practicing this are the following:

- Becoming acquainted with the process of death.
- Losing fear of death.
- Living physical life in a less restricted manner.
- Learning to look at death as merely a transition during which we shift our focus of attention from one place (the material plane) to another (the inner planes) and as a continuation of growth at different levels.

- Learning to better grasp the fact that the deeper core of existence is absolute, clear space and light.

The practice of the moment of death can be done alone or, ideally, with a support person close to us who can act as a guide during the practice and also during the actual moment of death if possible. To die in a state of devotion and prayer is a powerful force that can help the soul be catapulted toward higher states of consciousness. The ideal attitude would be that of being an observer as well as participant of the proceedings, without either trying to evade the process or identify with it.

1) <u>Lie down</u> on your back or your right side relaxed with closed eyes.
2) Have the <u>support person sit or kneel</u> beside you.
3) <u>Entertain positive thoughts,</u> focusing on higher consciousness, which can be represented either by a concept, such as love, or by the image of a beautiful place or enlightened person.
4) <u>Breathe calmly and rhythmically.</u> Inhale deeply then <u>while exhaling make the sound "AAAHH...."</u> This has a releasing effect and helps in letting go of everything. Focusing on the breath helps diminish any tension, worry, or fear, as well as disengage the etheric body from the physical body.

    The <u>support person breathes in synchronicity</u> with the dying person and <u>encourages</u> them to <u>make the sound "AAAHH..."</u> and <u>remain focused only on</u> breathing. Then the support person <u>gives commands,</u> either verbally or telepathically, like <u>"Easy, let go now"</u> or <u>"Now is time for letting go of everything,"</u> and <u>"Relax, release everything from your mind."</u>

    The <u>support person</u> conveys to the dying person a sense of tranquility, acceptance, and reassurance by <u>repeating commands</u> such as "Relax," "Be calm," "Let go," <u>"It is all right to leave,"</u> "Feel secure," <u>"Feel protected," "See and accept everything as yourself."</u>

    Achieving a relaxed state is fundamentally important to facilitate letting go and to open the mind to suggestions.
5) <u>Call a Master</u> or spiritual teacher of your choice, <u>sustain in your mind the highest possible ideal</u> for yourself, such as devotion, love, spiritual expansion., oneness with the Master, or oneness with God and <u>pray for your purification.</u> You may <u>repeat affirmations</u> like "I

am love," "I am one with God," "I am God," or "I am spirit."

The support person helps by calling the Master and reminding the dying individual to pray and repeat the above phrases.

6) Confront the stages of withdrawal of consciousness and dissolution of the inner elements in the following manner:

- Inhale deeply and imagine that you are pulling energy up from your feet, legs, and lower trunk toward your head. You may see this energy as a ball or a flow of white light.
- Exhale and see the energy flowing out of your head forming a circle down to the earth and then entering through your feet again. Make a full circuit of energy.
- Continue breathing in this manner and feel the bulk of your energy moving toward your heart.
- The support person directs the dying individual to breathe as described above.
- The support person gives the command to "Listen with full attention."
- The support person gently touches the First Chakra and says: "Allow yourself to lose strength and fall," "Remain awake," "Remain calm," "Do not be afraid of visions and sounds, for they are part of your mind," "Your Master is here with you."

This is the stage of earth dissipating into the next inner element of water.

- The support person gently touches the Second Chakra and says: "Allow yourself to be carried away by water and flow with it " "Remain awake," "Remain calm," "Do not be afraid," "Your Master is here with you."

This is the stage of water dissipating into fire.

- The support person gently touches the Third Chakra and says: "Allow yourself to burn and embrace the fire," "Remain awake," "Remain calm," "Do not be afraid," "Your Master is here with you."

This is the stage of fire dissipating into air.

- The support person gently touches the Fourth Chakra and says: "Allow yourself to fly and let go," "Remain awake," "Remain calm," "Do not be afraid," "Your Master is here with you."

This is the stage of air dissipating into ether, or consciousness.

7) The <u>support person encourages</u> the dying individual to <u>merge with the Master</u> by saying: "Become one with your Master."

8) The <u>focus of attention</u> should be on the <u>Fourth, or Heart Chakra.</u> The bulk of energy is concentrating at the heart level and the lower body feels numb, nonexistent, while the heart area feels expanded, throbbing, or experiences a sensation of pressure.

   The <u>support person</u> keeps <u>calling attention to the Heart Chakra</u> by saying: <u>"Stay in your heart."</u> Then, the support person <u>guides</u> the dying individual to the first <u>encounter with the Light</u> by helping them anticipate it and to bring their attention to it. The <u>support person says:</u> "Be calm," "Watch for the Light," "It is all right to go to the Light," "Be the Light," "You are the Light."

9) The <u>support person</u> starts <u>chanting a mantra, saying prayers, repeating affirmations, repeating the name of God or of a Master,</u> or simply <u>visualizing a Master.</u> Examples of these are: "OM" or "AUM," "OM MANI PADME HUM," "CHRIST AND I ARE ONE," "BUDDHA AND I ARE ONE," "ALLAH AND I ARE ONE," "KRISHNA AND I ARE ONE," "GOD AND I ARE ONE," "I AM SPIRIT," "I AM SOUL"

   This practice helps the dying person to have a positive and peaceful attitude and to remain focus on higher aspects of consciousness.

10) <u>Go through the stages of ejection of consciousness</u> in the following manner:

    • <u>Inhale</u> deeply and <u>imagine</u> that you are again <u>pulling energy upward,</u> this time from your heart toward your head.

    • <u>Exhale</u> slowly and <u>visualize</u> the <u>energy coming out of the top of your head</u> then <u>circling down to your heart</u> before once more ascending to your head. Continue forming a <u>constant circuit;</u> with each breath pull up a bit more of energy.

    • Remain breathing like this and <u>feel the core of energy moving to your head</u> this time.

    • The <u>support person guides</u> the dying person to breathe in this fashion.

    • If you lose your focus, the <u>support person tells you:</u> "Stay awake," "Be calm," "Continue breathing upward," "Your Master is here with you."

- At this point, the energy concentrates at the level of the throat. The <u>support person gently touches the Throat Chakra and massages it</u> with upward strokes while <u>chanting</u> "OM" or "AUM."

- Maintain your <u>focus at the top of your head</u> or even <u>above it</u> then <u>invoke and visualize</u> the Light or a Being of light.

- Now, your physical body and senses are completely gone and you may experience a sensation of <u>floating in space.</u> The <u>core of energy</u> is felt <u>behind the eyes,</u> pulsating, distending, and trying to rush out. With <u>each exhalation let go</u> and <u>allow yourself to expand and feel joy.</u>

- The <u>support person gently touches</u> the <u>Third Eye Chakra</u> and <u>massages</u> it upward while <u>saying:</u> "Stay awake," "Be calm," "Allow yourself to expand," "Be happy," "Your Master is here with you."

- Now you <u>eject yourself</u> out and upward through the top of your head. Inhale and then <u>exhale</u> while you <u>visualize your soul,</u> or energy, as a <u>white letter A</u> or as a <u>white light streaming out</u> of the top of your head like a fountain. <u>Feel yourself as light</u> attracted by Light, as being vacuumed into the cosmos.

- The <u>support person gently touches the Crown Chakra and says:</u> "Stay awake," "Be calm," "Do not be afraid," "Let go," "Visualize your soul as a white A or as a white light and eject it out," "Be one with your Master." The <u>support person visualizes the soul,</u> or consciousness, of the dying individual <u>being ejected.</u>

- <u>The soul breaks apart</u> and is liberated from the physical body. The dying person may experience it as being a <u>light energy rushing at unbelievable speed through a long corridor or tunnel,</u> as being suddenly catapulted with a tremendous velocity, which may cause a tendency to faint. The ideal situation is for the dying person to <u>remain in the center</u> of the tunnel and <u>focused on the bright white light at the end,</u> ignoring other dimmer lights that may appear at the periphery, to <u>abandon all thoughts and emotions</u> other than that of totally letting go of the mundane things connected to the former life, and melt into the Light. If the individual succeeds in doing so, the experience becomes one of <u>tremendous happiness</u> and a <u>sense of freedom and expansion.</u> This ideal experiences cause the individual's frequency to increase significantly so as to encounter the Light or Being of light in a state which more closely approximates Its higher frequency without resistance, and with complete trust.

- The <u>support person</u> aids by: <u>Repeating</u> "Stay awake," "Be calm and trust," "Stay in the center," "Be open and happy," "Recognize the Light as yourself," "Go to the Light and be the Light," "Melt into the Light."

<u>Invoking</u> the spiritual teachers of the dying person's choice and <u>imagining</u> that the rays of light emanating from the teacher are cleansing the dying individual. <u>Praying</u> for purification, protection, and guidance for the dying person.

<u>Imagining</u> themselves accompanying the dying person toward the Light.

11) The <u>support person keeps reminding</u> the departed one: "Do not be afraid," "All visions and sounds are part of yourself," "All visions and sounds are in your mind," "Your Master is with you."

12) The <u>support person invokes</u> Masters, spiritual guides, relatives, or friends of the departed person to help and guide the individual at the gates of the inner worlds.

If this practice is done repeatedly before the moment of death, the dying individual and the support person will be able to automatically do it at the actual moment of physical death, even in circumstances of a sudden, unexpected death. If at the moment of death the support person cannot be present, that person can still guide the departed individual after learning about the occurrence of death.

Practicing thus greatly increase our chances of being fearless, calmer, and more conscious at the time of death.

<u>Summary of the Steps to Follow at the Moment of Death.</u>
1) <u>Lie down</u> on your back or right side with the <u>support person kneel-</u>

ing beside you.

2) Have an <u>attitude</u> of acceptance and of being an observer.

3) <u>Focus your mind</u> in positive thoughts, or on a Master of your choice.

4) <u>Make your breathing</u> calm and rhythmic. <u>Exhale</u> with the sound "AAAFIH..." The <u>support person breathes</u> in unison and <u>directs the breathing</u> of the dying person. The <u>support person says:</u> "Relax," "It is time to let go," "Release everything from your mind," "Be calm and secure," "It is all right to leave," "You are protected."

5) <u>Invoke a Master</u> of your choice and try to <u>sustain a feeling</u> of devotion, love, and oneness with the Master or with God.

   <u>Pray</u> for your purification or <u>repeat affirmations</u> such as: "I am love," "I am spirit," "I am one with the Master," "I am one with God," "I am God." The <u>support person</u> invokes the Master and <u>reminds</u> the dying individual to pray or repeat the affirmations.

6) With your breathing and consciousness <u>create a full loop of energy</u> moving continuously from your feet to your head, then down to your feet again. <u>Feel the bulk of your energy</u> moving upward toward your heart. The <u>support person directs</u> this breathing.

7) The <u>support person says:</u> "Listen with complete attention," then <u>touches the first chakra and says:</u> "Allow yourself to lose strength and fall," "Remain awake," "Remain calm," "Do not be afraid of visions and sounds, for they are part of yourself," "Your Master is with you" (dissolution of earth into water.)

8) The <u>support person touches the second chakra and says:</u> "Allow yourself to be carried by water and flow with it," "Remain awake," "Remain calm," "Do not be afraid," "Your Master is with you" (dissolution of water into fire.)

9) The <u>support person touches the third chakra and says:</u> "Allow yourself to burn and embrace the fire," "Remain awake," "Remain calm," "Do not be afraid," "Your Master is with you" (dissolution of fire into air.)

10) The <u>support person touches the fourth chakra and says:</u> "Allow yourself to fly and let go," "Remain awake," "Remain calm," "Do not be afraid," "Your Master is with you," "Merge with your Master" (dissolution of air into ether.)

11) <u>Feel your energy</u> in your heart, <u>visualize</u> a Master or the Light and <u>repeat</u> a mantra, or affirmation such as "OM," or "AUM," "OM

MANI PADME HUM," "I am soul," "I am spirit," "I am one with Christ," "I am one with Buddha," "I am one with Allah," "I am one with Krishna," "I am one with God."

12) The support person says: "Stay in your heart," "Be calm," "Watch for the Light," Go to the Light," "Be the Light," "You are the Light."

13) The support person chants: "OM," "AUM," or "OM MANI PADME HUM."

14) Following your breath create a smaller loop of energy moving from your heart to your head, then out and back to your heart.

15) The support person guides this breathing and says: "Stay awake," "Be calm," "Continue breathing upward," "Your Master is with you." Feel the energy in your throat and visualize your Master.

16) The support person touches the Throat Chakra and massages it upward chanting "OM," or "AUM."

17) Move your focus to the top of your head or above it, invoke and visualize the Light or a Being of light and feel the energy in the eyes.

18) The support person touches the Third Eye Chakra and massages it upward saying: "Stay awake," "Be calm," "Let yourself expand," "Be happy," "Your Master is with you."

19) Visualize your energy or soul as a white light or a white letter "A" and project it out of the top of your head with each exhalation. Feel yourself expanding.

20) The support person touches the Crown Chakra, visualizing the soul of the individual being ejected out, and says: "Stay awake," "Be calm," "Do not be afraid," "Let go," "Visualize your soul as a white light and eject it out," "Be one with your Master."

21) Feel yourself moving at a tremendous speed through a long corridor. Stay in the center. Focus on a bright light at the end. Feel free and happy. Merge with the Light.

22) The support person says: "Stay awake," "Be calm and trust," "Stay in the center," "Be open and happy," "See the Light as yourself," "Go to the Light," "Be the Light."

23) The support person invokes the spiritual teacher, prays for the purification, protection, and guidance of the dying individual, and imagines walking the dying person to the Light.

24) The support person says: "Do not be afraid," "All visions and sounds are part of yourself," "All visions and sounds are in your

mind," "Your Master is with you."

25) The <u>support person invokes</u> Masters, spiritual guides, relatives, or friends of the dying individual to help the departed from now on.

CHAPTER VI

Help for the Dying and the Living

Psychological and Emotional Stages when Facing Imminent Death
According to Dr Elisabeth Kubler Ross, individuals who are given news about their inevitable death experience certain emotions and mental states in a specific sequence, those who are close to the dying individuals also go through a similar sequence of reactions as listed below:

Dying Individuals	Persons Close to Dying Individuals
-Shock and astonishment	-Shock and astonishment
-Denial and withdrawal	-Denial and resistance
-Emotions of: indignation, resentment, affliction, anguish, envy, anxiety, and dread	-Emotions of: indignation, resentment, affliction, anguish, envy, remorse, and embarrassment
-Negotiating to obtain either release from pain, strength, or prolongation of life in exchange of praying and promising God something	-Negotiating to obtain either release from pain, strength, prolongation of life in exchange of praying and promising God something

- Despondency and hopelessness due to a sense of failure and deprivation

-Despondency and hoplessness due to a sense of loss

- Guilt about unfinished business, financial problems, or abandonment of loved ones

-Shame because of past actions

-Finally acceptance

-Finally acceptance

Support and Aid before the Moment of Death

Generally, the best people close to dying individuals can offer is to help them have a good death, which means to die without distress, easily, peacefully, and as conscious as possible. Of primordial importance is to take amorous care of dying individuals at all times. The following are practical actions that can help significantly dying persons to feel better.

1) Speak the Truth

We should never lie, or distort the truth, nor be evasive to dying individuals. If we are not sincere, we only cause them further despair and isolation, for at a deep level they know the reality of what is transpiring. Thus we should speak the truth about their imminent departure, although we should do it when we sense they are willing to hear. We must do it calmly, with care, and with emphasis on death as an inherent part of life.

Being direct and speaking the truth to dying individuals will allow them to take advantage of the opportunity to prepare themselves to face reality, reflect on their life and its purpose and to discover their own strength and commanding capacity.

2) Listen Attentively

Affectionately encourage the dying individuals, making them feel at ease and free to communicate their inner thoughts and emotions facing death. Listen attentively, with calmness and compassion. Do not interrupt them or minimize what they are telling you. Make them feel that they are regarded with acceptance, without judgment. Help them reveal their worries, fears, sorrow, and depression so that they can eventually conquer them. Also help them see their abilities so that they can use them as strengths in facing death.

3) Acknowledge Them as They Are
We should accept dying individuals unconditionally, with all their various character traits and circumstances of their life stories.

The process of dying usually brings negative and suppressed emotions to the surface or causes a numbness of emotions. So we may have to deal with a totally uncommunicative and withdrawn person, or on the contrary, we may face individuals who express anger, impotence, grief, envy, or guilt. We may even become the object of their blame or of the release of their negativity. We must be prepared not to take anything personally, be patient, and show them understanding, making them feel that we are there for them and that what they are feeling is only natural under the circumstances.

Further, dying individuals should be helped to regain peace and should be permitted to disengage from their relationships and their physical life in the manner they wish. We may need to ask them what it is that they need the most from us to help them.

4) Demonstrate Unconditional Love
We should see dying individuals as our equals and not be judgmental or feel sorry for them, instead showing our compassion and love in a relaxed and genuine manner. We need to empathize with them so they feel comforted, reassured, and empowered individuals. If we place ourselves in the shoes of a dying person and feel what we would need to be comforted, then we can offer exactly that to the person that we are trying to help.

5) Establish Direct Physical Connection
We can alleviate the feeling of loneliness that dying individuals may experience by gently touching them, embracing them, holding their hands, maintaining eye contact, massaging them, or breathing in unison with them, all of which can be beneficial to them. These simple actions turn out to be extremely important and significant for a dying person.

6) Cautiously Use Humor
Using humor with dying individuals, always with sensitivity, can relieve tension and feelings of sorrow or depression, thus helping to make the environment

more uplifting and the dying individual maintain a positive attitude at the moment of death.

7) Assist Them Accepting Death

We can assist dying individuals in better accepting death by helping them feel the sacredness of the moment and understand the fact that death is only part of life. We must help them to know that in truth there is no death and induce them to feel love, consecration, and trust. We can also show them that voluntarily relinquishing their life to the superior will of God can bring them strength, serenity, and command over the situation.

8) Help Them be Optimistic and Hopeful

We can help the dying be optimistic and hopeful by encouraging them to see the positive goals they have attained in their recent life, feel glad about that, and focus on their goodness remembering their true essence of spirit and higher nature.

9) Stimulate Their Joy

We can stimulate the joy of dying individuals by helping them to reach deep inside those seeds of happiness that we all possess. We do this simply by making them remember joyful moments of their life, or practice meditation.

10) Guide Them to Discover Inner Strength

We can guide dying individuals to discover inner strength and their own source of healing by encouraging them to meditate, pray, and invoke beings of light to help concerning their circumstances. Totally being there and giving them full attention we can also set a good example by exuding love, confidence, and calmness ourselves thus modeling inner strength for them.

11) Help Them to Take Care of Unfinished Business

We can help dying individuals take care of unfinished business by assisting them in liquidating material matters and releasing emotional and mental burdens, such as feelings of resentment and guilt, involving others and themselves. We should guide them to sincerely ask for cleansing and purification. Also we can encourage them to ask forgiveness from others when necessary, as well as forgive themselves.

12) Encourage Them to Release Bonds and Depart

We can encourage dying individuals release bonds and depart by allowing them and their loved ones to freely express their sadness, openly demonstrate the love they feel, cry together and say farewell. Further, since dying individuals need to be given a sort of permission to die in peace and be reassured that loved ones left behind will be fine, they must be told by persons who are close to them that it is all right to leave and to do not be concerned about them.

The ideal situation would be that in which the dying individual completely let go external and internal attachments.

13) Assist Them with Spiritual Practice

We can assist dying individuals with the spiritual practice of their preference by doing the following:

- Encouraging them to recall their dreams and talk about them.
- Prompting them to say prayers, repeat mantras, or use positive affirmations.
- Encouraging them to meditate as an aid in realizing that the physical body is illusory so it is easier to let go of. It also helps such people comprehend the essence of the mind, which can be beneficial to better understand our condition after the transition of death.
- Guiding them to use visualizations, for example imagining a beautiful place where they are going or visualizing their melting into light or their Master. Also seeing the Master irradiating light that cleanses and heals them until they see themselves as light merging with the light of the Master.

All these practices, with the exception of working with dreams, can be done by the support person alone when dying individuals are unconscious.

14) Practice for the Support Person

The following practice, done by the support person, is helpful for the dying individuals to be relieved and maintain strength and serenity.

- Watch the dying person directly or imagine them.
- Feel compassion, open your heart, and breathe in all the suffering and fear of the dying individual.

- Breathe out, from your heart, light filled with love, joy, and peace to them.

Support and Aid at the Moment of Death

We can do several things to assist dying individuals at the moment of death to create an ideal situation for a good death. We must keep in mind that our behavior is crucial to helping the dying leave peacefully or die without fear or anxiety and not to delay their departure due to concern about situations on Earth.

The Environment

1) It is very important that the environment around the dying individual remains quiet, peaceful, and has a sacred ambience. Individuals present should contribute positively by remaining serene and silent, and maintaining a state of devotion with a positive attitude, since crying, feeling guilty, afraid, or angry may negatively affect departing souls by undermining their focus on death experiences, as well as negatively altering the qualities of these experiences. It is preferable, if possible, that individuals die at home, surrounded by intimate objects and persons, a circumstance that is less traumatic for the dying since it helps them to feel loved and protected.

2) It is ideal if people whom departing individuals love dearly are present at the moment of death, including children, for their energy may enliven the dying person and may help to create an elevated atmosphere. Also, children should be told the truth about the state of dying individuals and must be educated about the fact that death is a natural and sacred part of life itself

3) The place of death should be gladdened with flowers, plants, and photographs of lovely sites, or of people close to the dying.

4) Music, especially classical, or soft music can be an important aid to helping dying individuals release bonds with the physical plane and break free, as can reading poetry or spiritual subjects.

5) Burning incense, particularly sandalwood, which belongs to the energy of the First Ray of Creation, also facilitates breaking free from the physical body and eliminating obsolete patterns of energy. In the case of death, the First Ray's energy acts as a dismantling force for old energy patterns.

6) Placing an orange light somewhere in the room of dying individuals can help them focus on the head area and stimulate the brain centers which impulse the kundalini/shakti energy to ascend from the Root Chakra through the central channels during the process of withdrawal of consciousness.

7) Creating a small sanctuary in some corner of the room, where the sacred elements of earth, water, fire, air, and ether are represented and images of enlightened beings are displayed helps to build up a sacred atmosphere that can connect dying persons with larger cosmic principles.

8) Heartfelt prayers that focus on accepting the Will of God and ask for guidance for the departing individuals have the power to unify all the persons present and create a place of safety for the dying, as well as provide a state of peace and devotion. The same effect can be attained by reciting positive affirmations or chanting mantras.

9) Sending loving thoughts and beams of white light to departing individuals helps to dissipate negative energy and the persons feel supported and reassured.

10) Having a support person to guide dying individuals through the process of death is very important since this can minimize the dying individual's fear and maximize their control over the death experience.

The Dying Person

1) The dying person should avoid pharmaceuticals that may obscure consciousness and prevent the individual from fully experiencing the moment of death.

2) Ideally, according to Buddhist teachings, the dying person should lie down on the right side, the position in which Gautama Siddhartha, the Buddha, died, with the right hand positioned under the right check, obstructing the right nostril to block subtle channels of energy that may promote a misconception of reality. If possible, the head of the dying person should face east, thus honoring the direction that represents spirit. This posture helps the consciousness depart from the highest portal represented by the Crown Chakra, and facilitates the realization of the true nature of mind.

3) The ideal attitude for dying persons is calm openness while focusing

with mind and heart on spiritual teachings. It is very helpful for them to focus attention on a figure of light or Master, merging their mind with that of the Master as the death process proceeds.

The Support Person

1) The support person should have a clear understanding of the process of death as only being part of life, as well as of the sacredness of the moment and the opportunities it presents to the departing soul.

2) The support person should remain in a devotional state of consciousness, disengaging completely from their own emotions of grief, fear, or guilt, in order to help efficiently.

3) The mind of the support person should remain clear, calm, and loving so they can transmit strength and support to the dying individual, as well as effectively impart the necessary instructions and help the dying individual positively and peacefully face the extraordinary experiences that dying offers.

4) Through pure compassion and shearing, the support person should empathize with the dying person in order to provide them with an image of love and comfort.

5) The support person must be totally focused and observant, with heart and mind.

6) Rather than merely or impotently observing, the support person must feel invigorated by aiding to alleviate and empower the dying person.

7) The support person must become an unobstructed conductor of positive energy.

8) The support person should keep in mind their role as somebody who energizes, comforts, leads, and supports.

9) The support person should give directions and repeat positive affirmations during the death process using a serene, slow, and soft but resolute voice. The following is an example of positive affirmations the support person can repeat and guide the dying individual to think about at the moment of death:

    "My body is not me. I am not trapped in this body"

    "My eyes are not me. I am not trapped in these eyes"

    "My ears are not me. I am not trapped in these ears"

    "My nose is not me. I am not trapped in this nose"

"My tongue is not me. I am not trapped in this tongue"

"Emotions are not me. I am not trapped in these emotions"

"Thoughts and ideas are not me. I am not trapped in thoughts and ideas"

"This mind is not me. I am not trapped in this mind"

"Objects are not me. I am not trapped in objects"

"These forms are not me. I am not trapped in forms"

This practice helps to break free from identification with temporary bodies of manifestation and the physical sense organs.

10) The support person should remain by the physical body of the departed for one hour after clinical death to continue reminding the individual to do not be frightened and to merge with the Light.

Support and Aid after the Moment of Death

During the first thirty to forty days after physical death, the departed soul may still have bonds with the physical realm of existence and their recent life period. Throughout this period particularly they are likely to need our help, and it is possible to communicate with them. In the majority of cases, the individuals do not merge with the Light (Monad) and may be in a state of disorientation and strongly pulled toward the Earth plane. The nature of our help should be to guide them so they realize their new state of being and recognize the Light as themselves, and completely let go of fear, attachments to their former life, and reactions to what is going on at the mortuary, funeral and among the living left behind.

We can assist the recently departed in the following ways:

1) <u>With Our Attitude and Behavior</u>

We must remain mindful of the fact that our thoughts, feelings, and actions can strongly impact the consciousness of dead persons, pulling them back to the Earth plane, causing them conflict, or even hurting them, or, on the contrary, helping them to focus on their new tasks and advance in the spiritual realms. We must stay centered and balanced, encouraging them so they can adjust to their new circumstances in a positive and peaceful state of mind.

2) <u>Sending Positive Thoughts and Feelings</u>

We should send reminders for dead people to understand that they have transited to the inner worlds, not to try to return to the Earth plane but to surrender to their new existence, not be afraid, instead to focus on the new surrounding circumstances. We should also send them loving, peaceful thoughts, remind them to merge with the Light and that they may call for help from spiritual beings and masters.

Finally we should send wishes for their prompt realization of the new reality and their liberation from the astral body.

3) Talking to Them

We should attune ourselves to the dead person and talk aloud to them from our heart, telling them that we are all right, that we understand, that we love them very much, that we let them go and wish them well in their new mode of existence.

4) Reading

We may read passages from the Scriptures, spiritual teachings related to death, poetry related to death, or from *The Tibetan Book of the Dead* to help the departed navigate the stages after dead.

5) With Prayers

Our thoughts and words create focused energy that impacts on the astral body of the dead person and aids them with the dissipation of this body. Our prayers should be honest and loving, wishing for the dead individual to clearly see their path, do what is required of them, and ask for the available spiritual help.

6) With Invocation and Visualization

We can call upon a Master or a being of light to guide them. To do this, with all the strength of our mind and heart, we envision the pure light emanating from the Master engulfing the dead person, bringing compassion, love, peace, and purification to them, then we envision the dead person melting into the limpid light of the Master.

7) Repeating Positive Affirmations

Examples of positive affirmations include:

"Go to the Light"

"Merge with the Light"

"You are light"

"Feel the joy now"

"Feel the freedom"

"Feel the lightness"

8) Chanting Mantras

Examples are:

"OM", or "AUM"

"OM MANI PADME HUM"

9) Playing Music

We can play soft and melodious music, which helps the spirit to soar.

10) Making Offerings

We can donate the dead person's possessions to the needy, perform charitable actions in their name, or give money for a tree to be planted in their name.

11) Sponsoring

We can organize gatherings for prayers or spiritual practices in their name.

12) Practicing Meditation

We can invoke the dead person and dedicate our meditation to them in a state of devotion and compassion.

Support and Aid for Those Left Behind on Earth

We can help the families and close friends of a departed person to heal in the following ways:

— First, help them to understand that the dying individual is gradually becoming detached from them in preparation for death and that they must not resist letting go of the individual when the moment of dead arrives.

— Once the person has died, permit them to freely express any distressful emotions of anguish, resentment, despair, or guilt that surface. Support them so they can affront their feelings bravely and frankly. Teach them not to suppress their grief but instead to acknowledge and surrender to it without resistance. Make them understand that this feeling will definitely start to regress and decrease.

— Let them know that such emotions are natural and that they may experience them periodically for a long time. However, the pain and suffering eventually will cease. Then reassure them by saying that after their initial shock and painful awareness of the loss, they will experience a time of adjustment, and eventually recuperation and peace.

— Encourage them to forgive themselves and let go of their own negativity surrounding the dead and finally let go the dead person so they can peacefully continue their own life. Remind them that if they persistently hold on to the departed person in a possessive, or sad way they are actually harming that person by obstructing their necessary work in the inner realms of existence.

— Coach them to call for and speak to the dead person saying anything they want to say with complete honesty, then to let go of their own hurt feelings and the dead individual as well. Guide them to use the following instructions:

  • Imagine the departed one standing in front of you.
  • Intensely feel all your love and acceptance flowing to the departed one and feel their love and compassion coming to you.
  • Say good bye to the departed one and release the individual.
  • Visualize the person turning their back to you and going away.

— Encourage them to spend time in contact with nature, such as in the mountains, forests, country side, or near bodies of water and to release their pain into nature.

— Direct them to become engaged in physical movement and breathing exercises.

— Encourage them to use colors, fragrances, music, and reading to uplift their spirit.

— Advise them to pray for help, courage, fortitude, understanding, and blessings from enlightened beings.

— Explain to them how working with dreams and meditation may be helpful in healing.

— Remind them that their life has a meaning and a purpose of extreme value, interrelated to the whole of existence and sacredness of life. Thus they should channel their energy into productive and joyful endeavors.

— Advise them to do something positive in the name of the departed, such as doing something the dead person would have liked to do; completing something the dead individual could not finish while alive; dedicating prayers or meditation to the dead person; or vowing to live a more purposeful, more aware life as a result of the dead person's influence.

— Finally, make them understand that the departed person will always be inside their heart and thus always with them, in mind and essence.

CHAPTER VII

Summary of the Process of Death and Cycle of Reincarnation

The summary of the process of death and cycle of reincarnation in this chapter provides a quick review of the significant stages of events regarding death already discussed in greater depth in previous chapters.

1) Preliminary Signs of Death

   There can be many preliminary signs of death, depending on the health, circumstances of individuals, and their degree of awareness.

2) The Moment of Death or Restoration Stage

   The individual disengages from the physical body and the consciousness, or soul, departs. Dissolution of the inner elements occurs, chakra by chakra, corresponding to particular physical symptoms as well as visual and audio phenomena. The ideal responses would be:

The dying person	The support person or guide
Be calm and fearless.	Be calm and balanced.
Entertain positive thoughts.	Entertain positive thoughts.
Invoke a master or deity.	Invoke a master or deity.
Repeat a mantra or an affirmation.	Describe the dissolution of the

Recognize the phenomena as projections of the mind.	inner elements and gently touch each chakra.
	Encourage the dying individual not to be afraid and to remain peaceful.
	Repeat a mantra or an affirmation.

3) ## The First Review of the Recent Life
At this point, a quick replay of important scenes of the recent life occurs.

4) ## First Encounter with the Light
The breath ceases, and clinical death is declared. The consciousness, or soul, is within the central channels of energy at the level of the heart chakra, and encounters the Light for the first time. The person may then be in shock, or extreme awe, or in panic and retreat, faint into unconsciousness, or merge with the Light, the naked true nature of the mind, in various degrees. The ideal responses would be:

The dying person	The support person or guide
Be calm, fearless, and awake.	Be calm and balanced.
Recognize the Light as the self, letting go of everything else and merging with it.	Direct the dying person to not be afraid and to recognize the Light as the true nature of the mind and merge with it.
Chant a mantra.	Chant a mantra.

5) ## The Soul's Exit from the Physical Body
The soul's exit from the body usually takes place through one of the three portals: the solar plexus chakra, the heart chakra, or the head chakras, depending on the circumstances. Shortly after exiting the physical body, the soul also casts off the etheric body. The silver cord, or magnetic energy cord, breaks, signifying that the last magnetic attraction

between the dense physical body and the other bodies and soul is gone. The etheric body remains for a while near the physical body and then disintegrates. The soul is now only clothed with the emotional, or astral body, and the lower mental body. The soul goes through the tunnel experience, facing the revelation of different aspects of the mind (mental energy released in the form of visions, lights, and sounds), the second encounter with the Light (its own Monad), some sort of questioning, and the second life review. At any of those moments the dead person can recoil in fear, fall into unconsciousness, or experience true recognition of the Self and merge with the Light, emerging out of duality. The ideal responses would be:

The dead person	The support person or guide
Be calm, balanced, and fearless.	Be calm and balanced.
Remain in the center of the tunnel. Let go of everything. Recognize visions, lights, and sounds as reflecting the contents of the mind. Recognize and merge with the Light.	Guide the departed person to stay in the center of the tunnel, to not be afraid, to let go of everything except The Light at the end of the tunnel, to recognize the visions, minor lights, and sounds as reflecting the mind's contents, and to merge with the Light.

6) Encounters and Realizations

The soul encounters relatives and friends who have already died and also spiritual guides and helpers. The dead person realizes that individuality still exists, some kind of body still remains, communication is telepathic, perceptions are more vivid and clear than in the recent life, and feeling, thinking, and reasoning are still possible. The individual feels lighter and less restricted. The ideal responses would be:

The dead person	The support person or guide
Be calm and awake.	Be calm and balanced.
	Guide the departed person to not be afraid and remain calm.

7) Invigoration of de Soul, Rearrangement of the Emotional Body, and First Slumber of the Soul

The energy of the soul is strengthened by the energy of spiritual guides. During the slumber of the soul the individual experiences a slower review of the recent life to reflect on and integrate experiences and learning, purification, letting go, focusing attention on the spiritual worlds, and adjustment to the new circumstances waiting on the astral plane. The ideal responses would be:

The dead person	The support person or guide
Be calm and awake.	Be calm and balanced.
Be open to receive the energizing force. Let go of attachments.	Send loving thoughts to the departed.
	Practice prayers and meditation.

8) Awakening in the Astral Plane

The individual becomes conscious on the appropriate sub plane of the astral world, corresponding to the vibrations of the outermost layer of the individual's emotional body according to the individual's degree of development. The ideal responses would be:

The dead person	The support person orguide
Remain calm and aware.	Be calm and balanced.
Ask for help and guidance.	Send loving thoughts to the departed.
Take advantage of the opportunities for further learning.	Practice prayers and meditation. Talk to the dead person to help them to accept the new situation.

9) First Appearance before the Karmic Council (fourth life review)

The individual appears before the Karmic Council, the purpose of which is to help and support the individuals in their evolution and realization of the Divine Plan, always operating in accord with the universal Law of Karma, a balancing mechanism and corrective teaching device but not a punitive measure.

10) Life in the Astral Sub-planes or Shedding Stage
Individuals reunite with their spiritual families. During this period, the individual works on residues of passion, feelings, and desires, pursuing the same interests that the person exhibited during the recent physical life. The individual still retains the predominant features of the last personality on Earth. Later the person regains memory of the personalities of past lives. Also during this time the individual continually evaluates past lives to successfully integrate acquired experiences. It is a time of gradually shedding the emotional or astral body, of extensive learning, and of evolution with the help of guides and teachers. It could even be a time used to help others in need.

In general, this is a period of healing, purification, integration, restoration, and consolidation, although less evolved individuals are not fully conscious of this process. Each person here will be confined within conditions determined by their own level of evolution.

11) Second Death and Second Slumber of the Soul
A considerable part of the desire nature of the individual has been lived out, thus the emotional or astral body is totally shed (second death) and now the person shifts the focus of attention toward the mental worlds. The person again falls into a state of unconsciousness, the second slumber of the soul, for purposes of rest and adjustment.

12) Life in the Lower Sub-planes of the Mental Plane (continuation of the shedding stage)
The individuals, in accord with their degree of evolution, may or may not awaken in the lower sub-planes of the mental plane. If the individual regains consciousness, life here involves working with the nature of the mind including the purification of thoughts from emotional stains, the modification of faulty believes and the letting go of old, rigid patterns of thought. As a result, the moral and spiritual character of the individual is developed. The more individuals advance at this time, the greater their sense of peace and joy. In the process, the lower mental body is consumed and discarded.

1 3) <u>Ascending to Higher Levels of the Mental Plane</u> (consolidation stage)
The soul is now free in its own world, in a state of contemplation, communion, and bliss, working with higher mind principles and noble ideals for the future.

14) <u>Sensing the Call for Rebirth or Reincarnation</u>
The soul becomes ready for a new period of action in the physical world, or reincarnation, feeling the pull of still unsatisfied ambitions and the need to balance former karmic debts. The soul is then guided toward reincarnation, either consciously or unconsciously.

15) <u>Second Appearance before the Karmic Council</u>
The Karmic Council, constituted by the Lords of Karma, must approve the new incarnation, since they determine the number of individuals allowed to exist in physical life at a given time in the history of a planet. Also they must examine the accumulated individual karma in order to assign the portion to be balanced in the coming life period, as well as choose the most appropriate embodiment that will provide the best opportunities to work on the allotted karma, to learn more, to express abilities, and to accomplish the mission of that life. Finally, the Karmic Council must evaluate the historical era of the planet to make sure its conditions serve the evolutionary needs of the individual.

16) <u>Preparation for Reincarnation</u>
The individual meets with spiritual companions, guides, and teachers to be advised and assisted in the preparation of the new life plan, if the person is sufficiently conscious and advanced to make choices and participate in the planning process.

Parents, geographical location, historical time, and gender are determined. The karma to be worked on is discussed, as well as what individuals, with whom the person has karmic links in need of balance, will be living during that period. In addition, a general delineation of the tasks to be accomplished, the personal goals, main lessons to be learned, contribution to society, and special mission for the individual's life are also arranged.

17) <u>Preparation of the Etheric Blueprint for the New Physical Body</u>
The etheric blueprint for the individual's new physical body is created
under the supervision of the Lords of Karma. Also the body elemental
and the guardian angel are summoned.

18) <u>The Descent of the Soul</u>
The individual soul retraces the journey through the mental and astral
planes. The permanent atoms are activated at each level; the permanent life atoms are attracted, as well as the substance from each plane
that will form the new lower mental, astral, and etheric bodies of the
individual.

   The soul establishes a close contact with the future parents, especially with the mother to be. The new etheric body is placed in the
mother's womb. Spirit works on the germ cells of the parents, resulting
in conception. An etheric womb is formed around the embryo, and the
soul makes strong energetic connections with it.

19) <u>The Work of the Body Elemental</u>
The body elemental and the builders of form, construct the new physical
body of the individual based on the model of the etheric body and directly influenced by the incarnating soul and the energies of the Law of
Karma.

20) <u>The Third Slumber of the Soul</u>
In preparation for appearance in the physical world the soul again falls
in a state of semi-consciousness and forgetfulness, the third slumber of
the soul. During this time the soul works to assimilate and integrate
everything that has been learned during the intermission period. The individual refocuses mentally and prepares spiritually for reincarnation,
as images of the future life and its purpose appear intermittently to the
individual.

21) <u>Rebirth or Reincarnation</u>
The soul, now enshrouded with new mental, emotional, etheric, and
physical bodies, emerges once more into the physical world of existence
to awaken progressively and continue evolution.

Necessary Distinctions

It is important for us to understand the difference between <u>death</u> and <u>planetary ascension:</u>

What we call <u>death</u> is only a transition to a different state, from the physical plane to the astral and mental planes, where our evolution continues. The lower bodies are discarded, usually in a state of unconsciousness. We need to come back to the physical plane through reincarnations to continue our evolutionary process, with temporary loss of memory of the inner worlds each time we begin a new physical life.

We can view <u>planetary ascension</u> as a conscious and voluntary act of leaving the physical world once we have attained "enlightenment", to move toward higher levels of existence in a body of light. In this state reincarnation is no longer needed, since this part of the evolutionary process is completed; nonetheless evolution still continues at a different level. The individual in this condition has attained enlightenment and has unbroken memory and awareness. This is the end result of one of the human evolutionary cycles through spiritual growth and initiations.

Planetary Ascension can be accomplished in two different manners: what is known as <u>Etheric Ascension or Resurrection,</u> and what is known as <u>Physical Ascension.</u>

The first modality or <u>Etheric Ascension</u> happens near or right after the death of the physical body, once the individual has attained enlightenment. It is a resurrection in an ascended etheric body of light created at will. This body of light has a resemblance to a dense physical body. Resurrection implies returning to the place where we came from. This modality of Ascension is also known as <u>Astral/Etheric Ascension</u> and <u>Electronic Light Body Ascension.</u>

The second modality or <u>Physical Ascension</u> takes place while alive in a physical body, once the individual attained enlightenment. In this case, the physical body does not experience the process of death but is transformed into pure light as the individual reappears in a higher dimension of existence. This immortal body or spiritualized physical body is not subject to aging, disease, or death.

Thus, this kind of Ascension implies to accelerate and lift the cellular structure of the physical body into the higher frequency of light to attain the "rainbow body of light" which is luminous, brilliant, and fragrant.

This modality of Ascension is also known as <u>Spiritual Ascension, Translation,</u> and <u>Physical Immortality.</u>

Conclusion

With this knowledge about the process of death and reincarnation, we can make the following important concluding observations:

- In reality, there is no death, or destruction of the Self as spirit, but only eternal life.
- What we call death is just a movement, a transition to a different state of consciousness where our evolution and awakening process continues.
- Thus because death is a sacred moment of transition that presents us with opportunities to evolve and to eventually free ourselves from the cycles of reincarnation, it should be a reason for celebration instead of suffering.
- Currently, there is a great need to change the way we view and approach physical death.
- It is necessary that people be educated about the true meaning of the death process and how to navigate through it with calmness, clear understanding, confidence, and even joy.
- We must learn to help and assist others in passing through the portal of physical death in the best possible manner.

CPSIA information can be obtained
at www.ICGtesting.com
Printed in the USA
LVOW06s1546240316

480607LV00023B/51/P